LIFEPOINTS

LIFEPOINTS

THE INSTANT GUIDE TO THE GOODNESS IN FOOD

Peter Cox and Peggy Brusseau

BLOOMSBURY

Publisher's Note
LifePoints and the LifePoints logo are protected by international copyright, trade mark and service mark legislation and may only be used with the express permission of the proprietor, The Alta Vista Corporation Ltd.

The information in this book was correct to the best of the Editor's and Publisher's belief at the time of going to press. While no responsibility can be accepted for errors and omissions, the Editor and Publisher would welcome corrections and suggestions for material to include in subsequent editions of this book.

This book may include words, brand names and other descriptions of products which are or are asserted to be proprietary names or trademarks. No judgement concerning the legal status of such words is made or implied thereby. Their inclusion does not imply that they have acquired for legal purposes a non-proprietary or general significance nor any other judgement concerning their legal status.

This edition first published in 1995 by
Bloomsbury Publishing Plc
2 Soho Square
London, W1V 5DE

Copyright © by Peter Cox and Peggy Brusseau 1995

The moral right of the authors has been asserted

A copy of the CIP entry for this book is available from the British Library

ISBN 0 7475 1828 9

Typeset by Hewer Text Composition Services, Edinburgh
Printed in Britain by Cox & Wyman Ltd, Reading

IMPORTANT NOTE

If you wish to begin a diet programme, it is always wise to ask your doctor to confirm that there are no medical reasons why you should not undertake a change of diet. As the diagnosis and treatment of medical conditions are responsibilities shared between you and your medical advisers, neither the authors nor publisher of this book can accept responsibility for the individual consequences of dietary treatment based on the recommendations described herein.

The LifePoints system as described in this book has been created for use by healthy adults only. It does not apply to pregnant or lactating women, or to children. Women who are pregnant or lactating should not consider any weight-reduction diet until they have returned to a non-pregnant, non-lactating condition. A reduction in protein intake is emphatically not recommended for a woman who is pregnant or lactating, as the health of her child relies on both a higher protein and higher calorie intake during this time.

CONTENTS

QUICK START

If you want to get the LifePoints system working for you right now, here's how . . .

---

❶ Flick through the comprehensive list of foods until you find two or three which you'd like to eat during the day.

❷ Jot down their LifePoints and RiskPoints numbers. LifePoints are a measure of the food's health-enhancing nutrients. RiskPoints are a measure of the food's harmful ingredients. So, choose foods with a *high* LifePoints number, and a *low* RiskPoints number.

❸ Continue to add further foods from the list, choosing as widely as possible from the first four groups. Gradually adjust your diet: your total RiskPoints should *not* exceed 100; your total LifePoints *must* be greater than 100.

Now you know how easy the system is to use. Why don't you experiment with it for a few minutes, perhaps checking up on some of your favourite foods, and then read on to learn more about the world's simplest and most effective diet-planning system.

INTRODUCTION

WHY THIS BOOK MAY BE
THE BEST INVESTMENT IN YOUR
HEALTH YOU'VE EVER MADE

———

Dear Reader,
It is said that knowledge is power. If that's so, then you have in your hands one of the most powerful tools for personal health that you are ever likely to find.

Would you like to feel confident that you're eating the healthiest, life-protecting food and avoiding the worst?

✔   LifePoints can help you.

Would you like to stop 'binge' dieting and discover a truly healthy way of eating with which you can be comfortable – permanently?

✔   LifePoints can help you.

Would you like to be able to tell the difference between good food and bad at a glance?

✔   LifePoints can help you.

The fact is that Lifepoints can help you to achieve all these – and many more – wonderful goals. And let us tell you right away that if you've ever tried calorie-counting, the Life-Points system is *easier* – far easier. On the one hand, we

3

believe it's the world's simplest system for optimum nutrition and weight regulation. On the other hand, we are convinced that it is by far the most powerful way yet devised to directly compare one food against another, thus helping you find the very best foods to eat – forever.

There's one thing this book *won't* do, and that's try to sell you yet another fad diet. We're not going to insist that you eat pineapples all your waking hours. We're not going to promise you an instant cure for cellulite. Nor will we tempt you with thin thighs in thirty days. Books which made extravagant claims such as these were very popular a few years ago. If all you want is yet another nine-day wonder diet book, then *LifePoints* isn't for you. Such books should really be shelved under 'fiction' in bookshops because that's about how close some of them get to reality. If you're every tempted to buy one of those fad diet books, please remember that nine out of ten people who go on such diets end up quickly regaining most or all of the weight they lose. Even worse, scientific evidence is beginning to indicate that repeated dieting can dramatically increase your risk of suffering from heart disease, diabetes and other modern killers. *LifePoints* is not that kind of book – indeed, it makes such gimmick diets extinct.

And don't you just hate what the word 'diet' has come to mean? Say 'diet' to most people, and they'll immediately think you're talking about a weight-loss regime. What a perversion of meaning! As if the only point of eating (or to be more precise, *not* eating) is to try and lose weight. This is what we believe your 'diet' should do for you:

- It should provide you with an optimum intake of all the life-protecting, health-enhancing nutrients that nature provides for us.
- It should steer you away from dangerous, unhealthy or

unwholesome foods that imperil your health (obesity is one, but only one, result of an unhealthy diet).
- And, yes – it should be fun, tasty and so satisfying that it leaves you feeling contented and well nourished.

Those are the guiding principles behind the LifePoints philosophy. Beyond these key considerations we felt a compelling need to produce a simple system which would help just about anyone to eat a good healthy diet. Pick up virtually any food in the supermarket today, and you'll be bombarded with nutritional information on the label. Increasingly, food manufacturers are displaying more and more nutritional information on their products – indeed, the rules and requirements seem to grow more complex and demanding every year. But here's a strange paradox. While there's never been so much information available, it's never been more difficult to understand what it all means. We'd bet that not one consumer in a million actually uses all this data. And it's not surprising. Just consider some of the insurmountable obstacles you'd face . . .

- Nutritional information on food labels is often presented as the amount of vitamins or minerals present in 100 grams of the food. But people don't eat in neat, 100 gram servings!
- Just working out the calories in a serving is difficult enough . . . but have you ever tried adding up all the vitamins and minerals? Don't – unless you want to carry a portable computer around with you!
- Try solving this. Food 'A' has 0.6 milligrams of niacin in a serving, and 72 milligrams of vitamin C. Food 'B' has 1.2 milligrams of niacin per serving, and 5 milligrams of vitamin C. Now . . . work out which is the most nutritious food to buy . . . and good luck!

These problems are just the tip of a Titanic-sized iceberg. Whoever dreamt up the regulations for the nutritional labelling of food has clearly never been near a supermarket shelf, nor have they tried to actually *use* the barrage of information which food products are increasingly forced to display.

What all this labelling mumbo-jumbo conspires to do is very insidious. While appearing to give us increased nutritional information, it actually *deprives* us of effective control over the food we eat. Too much information – especially if it's almost incomprehensible and impossible to use – is just as bad as none at all.

So when we created the LifePoints concept we wanted to devise a way of measuring the good things, and the bad things, in a food so that you could use this information effectively. This, we hoped, would give you back control over your food intake – in a word, it would empower you. We knew that it was possible to create such a system, because we'd done it before. A few years ago, we wrote a book called *The Quick Cholesterol and Fat Counter*. It was the first book in the world to do something which a great many people had obviously been waiting for, and it became a best-seller. Until its publication, no book had ever tried to give its readers a simple and effective way of identifying which foods were good for cholesterol level, and which ones were bad. In fact, some experts told us it couldn't be done . . . and others told us it wasn't worth doing. In the course of our research for it, we interviewed dieticians and other health professionals whose attitudes sometimes appalled us. Some of them were prescribing diets for their patients which were way too high in fats and other undesirable foodstuffs. 'Why?' we asked them. 'Because our patients won't eat anything better,' they shrugged.

We disagreed. We had more faith in our readers than

the experts had in their own patients. We thought that most people would be delighted to eat a cholesterol-lowering diet – providing they were given a method of planning it for themselves. *The Quick Cholesterol and Fat Counter* wasn't a rigid diet, it was a flexible and simple tool for readers to use as creatively as they wished. We didn't prescribe – we described! And this is what we found: ordering someone to follow a rigid, predetermined diet is almost always a recipe for failure. But give them a system to plan their own diet, and they will almost always succeed.

And *did* they succeed! 'I feel I must write,' said one reader, 'to tell you of my success in reducing my cholesterol level after reading your book. I was informed by my doctor that I should reduce my level which was 6.3 millimoles per litre. I bought a copy of your book the next day. After six weeks my cholesterol level was tested again and incredibly it was found to be 3.87 millimoles per litre. My doctor asked how I had managed to effect such a dramatic reduction. I told him of your book of which he took a note and said he would recommend it to other patients.' Another wrote: 'After my father had a heart attack . . . I had a blood test which gave a level of 7.2 millimoles per litre . . . I found your books on the shelves of a local bookshop and bought them. My next test showed my cholesterol level down to 5.2 millimoles per litre.' And another: 'I was horrified to discover my husband's cholesterol level at 14.3 millimoles per litre. After years of trying to find out what the large "lumps" were on his elbows and knees, I suggested a cholesterol test as a last resort. I don't want to bore you with a long history, but I want to say that after following your book, the level was reduced to 7.2 in eight weeks WITHOUT MEDICATION.'

LifePoints takes this philosophy of empowerment – now

proven to be so effective – to its ultimate conclusion. Quite simply, *LifePoints* is the world's first easy-to-use guide to the goodness in food. It lets you compare one food with another and see which is better for you. It lets you scrutinise your present diet, and correct it if necessary. It lets you plan a permanently healthy way of eating, and lets you change it whenever you want to. It lets you tell the difference between good foods and bad. And that's something which no book has ever done before.

We wrote this book – and its companion, *The LifePoints Cookbook* – because we are increasingly dismayed by the confusion that exists about diet and health. Today, there is virtually no common disease that cannot either be prevented or considerably alleviated by nutritional means. For decades the world's medical and scientific journals have published thousands of epidemiological studies and intervention studies which have given us a unique insight into the health benefits of particular patterns of eating, individual foodstuffs and, indeed, specific nutrients. Unbelievably, this formidable body of scientific research is routinely ignored by much of the healthcare profession, some of whom seem to view nutritional medicine as a fringe heresy akin to devil worship. Peter expressed our feelings about this in an article in the British Medical Association's *News Review* magazine: '. . . it is truly shocking that this hard-won knowledge should be so consistently ignored. Isn't it time that your profession cast its prejudices aside . . . looked at the evidence – and got angry?'

Unfortunately, we anticipate that some health professionals will condemn *LifePoints* out of hand because it refutes the most cherished dictum of orthodox dietitians which states that 'there are no good foods or bad foods, only good diets and bad diets'. This notion pervades traditional dietary thinking and has probably contributed to more avoidable illness and suffering than any other fallacious theory in modern healthcare. It is increasingly obvious from decades of painstaking research that certain foods are good for our health and certain foods are bad for us. How do we define good and bad foods? It's really very easy. We define a 'good' food as one that contains an abundance of health-promoting nutritional factors, while containing none of the substances that scientific investigation has shown to be hazardous to health and longevity. A 'bad' food is precisely the opposite. In between these two extremes there is a whole spectrum of foods, some better than others. *LifePoints* is the first book in the world to analyse and categorise food like this.

Simply gathering the raw data for this book took many months, and processing the final LifePoints and RiskPoints totals was an immense computing task. All this work has had one single aim – to give you an astonishingly powerful yet simple way to plan, analyse and correct your diet. As such, it represents a quantum leap in healthy eating. We can promise you that once you've used the LifePoints system for just a week, it will permanently change the way you think about food; calorie counting will quickly become obsolete. For the first time ever, LifePoints gives you the big picture about the healthy and unhealthy aspects of your food intake. If knowledge is power, then you've just taken the first step towards power over your diet – forever.

Peter Cox
Peggy Brusseau
London

PART 1
BEYOND CALORIES

Have you ever tried driving your car with one eye shut? Imagine it. You're travelling down a busy high street, using all your concentration to avoid pedestrians, other cars pulling away from the kerb, children darting into your path, and a hundred and one other routine but critical hazards, with just one eye to guide you. If you want a short life, but an exciting one, it's the only way to drive.

The first thing you notice when you're one-eyed driving is that you can't reckon distances with any accuracy. It's impossible to judge precisely how far away people, objects and other vehicles are from you: an extremely hazardous situation for you, and for them. When everything you see is squashed into just two dimensions, your brain just doesn't have enough visual information to be able to guide you safely. How long do you think you'd survive in that dangerous two-dimensional high street? The odds against you are dauntingly high.

Close one eye and suddenly your world consists of just two dimensions. You can see the width of an object and its height, but you can only guess at its depth and therefore its distance from you. A dangerous game to play – we emphatically don't recommend it.

No one in his or her right mind would try to drive a car with one eye shut. Only a fool or someone with a death-wish would attempt it. But that's precisely how most of us go about choosing our food.

THE ONE-EYED DIETER

When you think about food, you think about calories. A fresh apple has about 80 calories. A tin of baked beans has about 300. A cheeseburger, about 600. And that's how we've been used to measuring the value of the food we eat . . . in terms of calories.

But calories are by no means a satisfactory gauge of a food's worth or importance to the human body and its well-being. What judgement can you truly make about a food that yields, say, 300 calories? Can you tell whether that food is good or bad for you? Is it a healthy food or a health hazard? Will it tend to fortify or weaken your state of health? How well does it fit into the rest of your day's diet? Is it going to make you put on fat or lose weight? Does it contain health-enhancing nutrients or disease-promoting antinutrients?

Just knowing a food's calorie yield cannot possibly answer any of these vital questions. And yet that's the only basis by which most of us have ever tried to assess the quality of the food we consume.

And what, in any case, is a 'calorie'? You may be surprised to find out. Unlike other nutrients in food, you can't isolate calories. Give an orange to a biochemist and after some jiggery-pokery in the lab, she'll be able to give you test-tubes with most of that orange's vitamin C and other nutrients neatly separated out. Not so the calories. That's because calories have no tangible existence on their own . . . you can't see them, you can't taste them and you certainly can't separate them from the food itself.

The word 'calorie' derives from the Latin, 'calor',

meaning 'heat', and that gives us a clue to the real role of the calorie. It is simply the name of a unit used to measure heat energy. One calorie was originally defined as the amount of heat energy required to raise the temperature of 1 gram of water from 14.5°C to 15.5°C. Pretty obscure, isn't it? Today, a calorie is defined in mechanical rather than thermal terms, so that one calorie equals 4.184 watt-seconds (or joules). Like inches, metres, pints and other units of measurement, the calorie is a useful measure when used properly. For example, it takes 80 calories to melt one gram of ice and 540 calories to boil one gram of water. Burn one gram of carbon and you'll release 7,830 calories. Run vigorously and you'll expend about 15,000 calories a minute (yes, we said '15,000' – if you find this a bit puzzling, read on). All interesting enough – but what does it tell us about the quality of our food? Not much.

Merely knowing the amount of heat energy locked up inside the food we eat isn't going to tell us much about that food's quality – or its impact on our health. Scientists have conventionally used something called a 'bomb calorimeter' to measure the calorie yield of a food. They take a portion of the food in question – say a slice of cheesecake – and seal it inside a container. The air is pumped out and oxygen is pumped in. Then, an electric spark ignites the oxygen and – bang! – the food burns and heat energy is released. The container is immersed in a water bath and by measuring the rise in the water's temperature it is possible to calculate the calorie yield of the food. It doesn't sound much like the human digestive system, does it?

In fact, this standard laboratory technique is imperfect. Not all the energy locked up in food is available to the human metabolic processes. Although humans have an astoundingly large surface area of digestive tract through which the nutrients in foods are absorbed – if you spread it out, it would be larger than a tennis court – we don't absorb *all* the nutrients in food, and we don't use *all* the potential heat energy locked up in foodstuffs. Real world systems, such as digestion, are always far more complex than laboratory models.

The calorie yield of a food, as approximated by the bomb calorimeter, tells us something about the amount of heat energy locked up inside a food, and nothing more. And by the way, just to complicate matters, a 'calorie' when used in connection with food usually means a 'kilocalorie', or 1,000 calories. Sometimes you'll see it written like this: 'kcal', and sometimes like this: 'Cal'. From now onwards in this book, we're going to follow the normal, although rather illogical, convention of saying 'calorie' when we really mean 'kilocalorie'. Well, no one ever claimed that nutrition was a perfect science . . .

So here you are, planning your diet. You're looking at food labels in the supermarket and all you can really do is to compare the calorie yield of one food with another. You pick up two cans – both labels show approximately the same calorie yield. Which one are you going to choose? With only one nutritional dimension to work with, you might as well flip a coin.

Take another scenario. Now you're getting really pro- fessional at this calorie-counting business and you've bought a calorie counter. You've decided to limit yourself to about 1,600 calories a day, so you diligently plan your day's food intake . . . calculator in hand, pencil and rubber nearby. And holy mackerel, is it hard work! Juggling all those portion sizes, searching for a food which you can just squeeze into the limit . . . and, let's face it, doing a bit of cheating, too. Finally, you've done it – 1,600 calories or thereabouts. But what have you *really* achieved? Have you assured yourself a good intake of all the essential vitamins? No! Have you made sure that your day's food intake is healthily low in fat? No! Have you achieved anything at all other than keeping your energy intake down to 1,600 calories? No!

Here's the bottom line. Calories are merely a one-dimensional measure of a food's worth. They can tell you about its energy yield, and no more. Using calories – and only calories – to plan a healthy diet is about as sensible as trying to drive down a crowded high street with one eye shut. You're simply not getting enough information to do the job properly.

IF THE ONLY TOOL YOU HAVE IS A HAMMER, ALL PROBLEMS BEGIN TO LOOK LIKE NAILS

It's not hard to understand why calories have loomed so large in our food consciousness in recent decades. The only dietary sources of calories are carbohydrates, proteins, fats and alcohol. If your combined calorific intake of these substances greatly exceeds the amount of energy you expend, then your body very sensibly stores the excess energy as fat. We say 'very sensibly' because this marvellous ability to store food energy efficiently is one of our most impressive biological characteristics. Humans are one of the most successful species to ever walk, swim or crawl over the surface of the Earth, and our phenomenally efficient energy storage system is surely one of the most important factors in our success. Did you know that we have more fat cells (adipocytes) in proportion to our body mass than virtually any other creature – only hedgehogs and whales have a greater proportion of fat cells in their bodies. Even animals which we traditionally think of as 'fatties', such as pigs, seals, bears and camels, all have proportionately fewer fat cells than we do. Far from being a curse, this high proportion of fat cells is actually a tremendous evolutionary advantage because it allows us to cope with the uncertainty of a variable food supply; we can smooth out the peaks and troughs. No food today? No problem! We can live off our fat.

Of course, most Westerners don't have that particular problem any more. For most of us, there are no days without food, only days when there's too much too easily available. And that's one reason why half the adult population of countries such as the United States and Britain are overweight. What was once a major biological advantage has suddenly and treacherously turned into a life-threatening problem. Today, humans are the only animal species to be so seriously menaced by obesity. No other species has as much excess body fat as we do, and no other species so regularly commits suicide by over-feeding.

Let's be painfully honest with each other and admit that the major cause of obesity really is over-eating. Yes, there are other factors which influence our tendency to gain weight, such as our genetic susceptibility, our mothers' diet before and during pregnancy, and whether or not we were breastfed when young. But mainly, we just chow down too heartily. A recent scientific experiment demonstrated this very convincingly. It was conducted at St Luke's-Roosevelt Hospital Center in New York, where the food intake of a group of 'diet-resistant' women and men were studied. The doctors measured all the calories these people took in and burned up and they found that their metabolisms were perfectly normal. The real problem was quite clear – they were simply eating too much. And they were fooling themselves about how much they ate; they were actually taking in twice as many calories as they believed. To make matters even worse, they were getting a lot less exercise than they believed, too. Dr Steven B. Heymsfield, head of the weight control unit at the hospital, commented: 'These people really cannot invoke some genetic cause as the only explanation for their obesity. The main reason they are overweight is that they are over-eating. Let's not blame it on something that it isn't.' Quite right.

Why do we over-eat? Here, we can be rather kinder to ourselves. In the main, the cause of over-eating isn't gluttony or greed. Once again, it's all to do with our species' ancient (and until recently) highly successful feeding strategies. Animals in their natural environment never die from over-eating – the greatest threat comes from starvation. Evidently, the best survival strategy is to eat whenever the opportunity arises because you never know where the next meal's coming from. That's why many of us *still* eat whenever we get the chance, even though our logical minds tell us that there is no conceivable likelihood of starving to death.

Remember, it has taken our species a mere 50,000 years to evolve from our pre-human forebears to the humans we are today. In evolutionary terms, 50,000 years is no time at all. Today, inside our twenty-first-century minds and bodies, there are the genetic remnants of creatures that existed many millennia ago – creatures which, by our own standards, were not even human. The appendix, the coccyx (tail bone), the webbing that still exists between our fingers – these and other physical clues indicate that our pre-human ancestry is still very much a part of our make-up. Although our human ancestors split from the ancestors of chimpanzees all of 7 million years ago, there is only a tiny (about 1.6 per cent) genetic difference between modern humans and chimpanzees, which just goes to show how slowly evolution takes place. And that's really at the root of most of our dietary problems.

S. Boyd Eaton, Marjorie Shostak and Melvin Konner are three scientists whose work has done much to enable us to understand the causes of the dietary problems we all face today. 'Here we are,' they explain, 'in the late twentieth

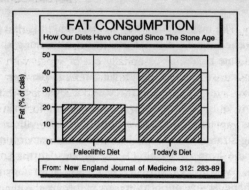

FAT CONSUMPTION
How Our Diets Have Changed Since The Stone Age

Fat (% of cals)

Paleolithic Diet   Today's Diet

From: New England Journal of Medicine 312: 283-89

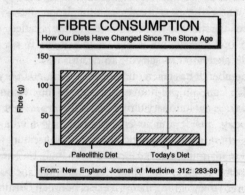

FIBRE CONSUMPTION
How Our Diets Have Changed Since The Stone Age

Fibre (g)

Paleolithic Diet   Today's Diet

From: New England Journal of Medicine 312: 283-89

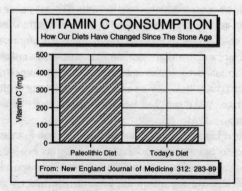

VITAMIN C CONSUMPTION
How Our Diets Have Changed Since The Stone Age

Vitamin C (mg)

Paleolithic Diet   Today's Diet

From: New England Journal of Medicine 312: 283-89

century, with a 40,000-year-old model body . . . adjusting as best we can to the complex demands of our lives. Yet with genetic make-ups essentially out of synch with our lifestyles, an inevitable discordance exists between the world we live in today and the world our genes "think" we live in still. This mismatch . . . can account for many of our ills, especially the "chronic diseases of civilisation" that cause 75 per cent of the deaths in industrial societies.' These same scientists have clearly shown that the Stone Age diet we are genetically programmed to consume differs in some vitally important ways from the type of diet most of us consume today. Some of the key differences are shown in the charts on page 18. You'll be pleased to know that the LifePoints system incorporates many features of the Stone Age diet – more about this later.

Sometimes our deep-rooted survival instincts are very effectively manipulated by major advertising interests. Take, for instance, the frequent and very prominent use of the word 'new' on many food products. Have you ever wondered why this word is featured so often on food packaging? The answer again lies in an old and once-useful behaviour pattern which we and other successful omnivores have evolved. Omnivores are animals that have adapted to eat a highly varied diet. Their successful survival strategy is continually to search out *new* types of food so that if one staple in the diet fails for any reason, there is always another food-source ready to replace it. What a great idea! But in nature, the urge to experiment with new food is carefully counterbalanced by the desire to be cautious. You can see both of these clever survival mechanisms demonstrated in the behaviour patterns of that other hugely successful omnivore feeder, the rat.

Rats, just like humans, are always ready to experiment with anything new. When a rat finds something unusual to eat (and like us, they are on the look-out all the time), she will carefully nibble a small amount, then leave it alone for some time. If she suffers no ill-effects in the meantime, she will return to the new food and may begin to include it in her diet. However, if the rat feels sick after eating that small sample of 'new' food, she will never eat it again. This is a highly successful technique, which frequently defeats the manufacturers of rat poisons. It is without doubt one of the most powerful feeding strategies of all time because it successfully reconciles two opposing imperatives: the ceaseless quest to find new food sources, and the urge to be cautious when faced with unknown danger.

We humans, too, use precisely the same technique. You can prove it for yourself – think back to a time when you felt ill soon after eating a particular type of food. It doesn't really matter whether your sick feeling was actually caused by the food you remember eating; what matters is that you now associate that food with an unpleasant feeling and, in all probability, will never eat that particular food again. It's in ways like this that our old survival mechanisms try to keep us away from food which may be dangerous for us. However, it's the other side of this mechanism – the strong instinct we all possess to experiment with anything 'new' – that gets us into so much trouble these days; there is simply so much temptation all around us. It is this constant desire to look for – and experiment with – new foodstuffs that makes us so vulnerable to regular over-eating.

With these immensely powerful instincts tempting us to 'Eat whenever you can!' and 'Try that new food right now!' it's hardly surprising that, in today's world of promiscuous consumption, many of us eat far too much. It's not that we're weak willed; it's just that we can't fight nature.

Once you begin to understand this, you'll appreciate why – in truth – we really don't have a calorie problem. We actually have something far more serious – a food strategy problem. And even more unfortunately, 'food strategy' is one of those things that comes hard-wired into our brains even before we're born. It's not something that's amenable to effortless modification.

The proof of this conclusion is all around us. Scientific data shows that the American male body mass index (a measure of obesity) has increased by 16 per cent over the last century, in line with increasing affluence and the ever-increasing availability of new, cheap and often unhealthy foodstuffs. Here's a rather more trivial, but equally telling, example: when New York's Yankee Stadium was built in 1922, the width of each seat was set to a generous 19 inches. Fifty years later, the average American posterior had broadened so much that the seats had to be widened to 22 inches. After thirty years of applied research into obesity, and a public expenditure of more than $100 billion in America alone, people are fatter than ever before.

Let's be quite clear about this – calling obesity a 'calorie problem' is about as sensible as calling an alcoholic someone with a 'pint problem'. In both cases, the units of measurement are being confused with the real cause. There's an old saying that goes: 'If the only tool you have is a hammer, all problems begin to look like nails.' We could update that to say: 'If the only tool you have is a calorie counter, every dietary problem begins to look like a calorie problem.'

And here's why that confusion matters so much: as long as we interpret obesity as being caused by 'an excess of calories', then the treatment for it will simply be to reverse the process, by trying to consume fewer calories. That process is called 'going on a diet'. Unfortunately, diets don't work.

Diets? Who Needs Them?

When you drastically reduce your calorie intake, your body thinks you're starving. As far as your body is concerned, dieting and starving are one and the same thing. Starvation is a life-threatening event which must have faced our species countless times in the past because the body already has an excellent survival strategy lined up, ready to be implemented at the drop of a calorie. The first thing it does is to lower your metabolism in order to conserve energy. The longer your food intake continues to be below what it expects, the harder your body tries to preserve that precious energy locked up as fat. That's why the first week of any diet produces an impressive result, yet subsequent weeks achieve little, if anything. Your body's deep-rooted instincts are fighting you all the way, and sooner or later, they'll win.

One particularly notorious way in which our instincts triumph over our will-power is through the binge impulse. Anyone who's ever attempted dieting will be familiar with it. You may know the scenario: your diet's lasted a few days and so far it's gone well. Then, in one insane and unrestrained moment, you find yourself behaving like a great white shark in a crowded swimming pool. Eat! Eat! Eat! As you maniacally bolt down everything that could possibly have a calorie or two associated with it, you start to feel helpless and guilty. How could you be so weak? How could you have ruined all your hard work in a momentary feeding frenzy? This sort of negative self-talk can sometimes lead to serious eating disorders such as bulimia.

But take it easy on yourself for a moment. When you think about it, the binge impulse is, yet again, a very logical and successful feeding strategy. Your body thinks that there is a severe food shortage which is causing you to starve. Trying to protect you, your instincts become super-sensitive to any potential source of food – and, of course, in today's society there are unlimited sources of food available everywhere. Drop your guard for just one instant, and the ancient survival instincts take over. If Freud were a dietitian, he'd say that the super-ego had been well and truly clobbered by the id.

And another thing – dieting is usually hell. You have to put up with absurdly small portions of your favourite foods, which requires super-human discipline, or an unhealthy streak of masochism. Even worse, you feel hungry most of the time, which makes you a real *kvetch* to your colleagues, friends and family. Ever wonder why dieters have to club together in those self-help groups? It's because nobody else wants to talk to them . . .

Joking aside, conventional calorie-restricted diets have even more serious drawbacks, too. Among the symptoms are:

- Bloating and distended stomach
- Constipation
- Depression
- Failure to produce collagen, the major protein of all connective tissues
- Feeling cold all the time
- Hair loss
- Headaches
- Lack of energy
- Loss of lean tissue
- Low blood pressure leading to dizziness
- Menstrual difficulties
- Sleep disruption
- Water retention
- Yeast infections

There are enough scientific studies around now for us to come to the certain conclusion that dieting, as it's usually practised, is ineffective in any long-term sense. In a 1986 Dutch study, men who experienced many stressful life events in a short period experienced a weight gain. That's not unusual; once again, it's our body's way of trying to protect us from harm. A year later, this weight gain had disappeared in almost all subgroups of these men. The exception was the subgroup that tried to lose weight by dieting; those who dieted had *gained* yet more weight. This study, reported in the *International Journal of Obesity*, makes no sense to those who believe weight gain is a 'calorie problem' which can be overcome simply by restricting calories. But when you see it in terms of a survival strategy, it makes perfect sense: those men had already been through a number of stressful life events, and the threat of starvation (i.e. dieting) seemed, to their bodies, to be just one more hazard. Their bodies actually responded splendidly by trying to conserve every last calorie.

Many scientific studies now confirm that if you want to put on weight, one of the very best ways to do it is to diet. Weight gain is particularly provoked by 'diet cycling' (continual diet/binge cycles), and it is such a well-accepted phenomenon that it is sometimes used in a clinical situation to help underweight patients put on bulk. How, precisely, does this happen? It's probably connected to the production of an enzyme called lipoprotein lipase (LPL) which is responsible for storing body fat. After starting a diet, LPL levels initially drop, then remorselessly rise again – sometimes to twenty-five times their normal level. The fatter you are to begin with, the more LPL you'll produce when dieting. This finding has been used to support the 'set point' theory of body weight regulation, which suggests that each person has an internal control system which predetermines how much weight, or fat, we should have.

If calorie-restricted diets worked effectively, there would be few people in the Western world with an obesity problem. In their recent paper entitled 'Diet and Health: Implications for Reducing Chronic Disease Risk', the Committee on Diet and Health of the National Research Council pointed out that 'food intake has declined over the past decade when body weight and presumably fat stores have, on average, increased'. In other words, our growing fatness cannot be explained by the fact that we're eating more calories – because we're not. Other studies have confirmed that Westerners today take in fewer calories than at the beginning of the twentieth century, while the level of obesity has stubbornly climbed.

We can draw three very important conclusions from all the evidence we've considered so far. First, merely knowing the heat yield of a foodstuff as measured in calories tells us next to nothing about its real nutritional worth to us. Second, conventional calorie-restricted diets have a very poor track record of success and often ultimately lead to weight gain. And third, since calorie-restricted diets don't work and since we're consuming fewer calories today than we used to but are getting fatter, we can reach the conclusion that effective weight control must involve more than just counting calories.

As you'll see, the LifePoints approach towards effective weight control is very subtle; you might call it 'the art of dieting without dieting'. We don't believe that crash diets are effective in the long run, nor are they necessarily safe for you. Neither do we believe that strict calorie counting usually achieves any worthwhile change. Instead, the focus of the LifePoints system is to trust our bodies and instincts a little more, while providing a helping hand and a system for developing and reinforcing our instinctive wisdom about the goodness and badness of our food choices. The LifePoints system can help you to regularise your weight by directing you towards eating good food and avoiding bad.

YES, THERE *ARE* GOOD AND BAD FOODS

Plain common sense tells most of us that some foods are indeed better for us than others. When the American Dietetic Association released the results of a recent public opinion survey into attitudes towards food, they found that three out of four people surveyed believed that there are 'good' and 'bad' foods. That finding must have vexed doctrinal dietitians everywhere because for years the profession has been telling us precisely the opposite – that virtually any food can be part of a 'well-balanced' diet.

Well, *someone* out there must be happily eating that legendary 'well-balanced' diet because we hear so much about it all the time. Someone out there must be eating all the burgers, all the french fries, all the ice cream and all the other high-fat foods we are so regularly told are fine for us 'when eaten as part of a balanced diet'. So far, however, we've never met such a person. All we see is evidence of people eating bad foods and becoming ill. Conversely, we see scientific studies following the health of people who eat good foods and they *stay* healthy.

Think critically for a moment about the myth of the 'balanced diet' and you'll soon realise just how preposterous it is. Here's how the myth goes: 'No food can be considered to be "good" or "bad" because virtually any food can be consumed provided it is eaten in the context of a balanced diet.' This means, for example, that burgers, fries and milkshakes are fine provided they are 'balanced' by the consumption of other foods. All right. But precisely what 'other foods'? That's never made clear. We can assume, however, that those mysterious 'other foods' contain the health-enhancing nutrients which burgers, fries and shakes lack. We can also assume that those 'other foods' *don't* contain the fats and other antinutrients that burgers, fries and shakes most certainly do contain. In other words, those 'other foods' are *good* foods.

Furthermore, foods such as burgers, fries and shakes contain absolutely no nutrients which can't be obtained from other food sources. Indeed, there are plenty of other foods that contain those nutrients found in burgers, fries and shakes, and which additionally *don't* contain the unhealthy fats and other antinutrient factors. So burgers, fries and shakes make no uniquely valuable contribution towards our overall nutritional health, but they do contribute several undesirable antinutrients that we could well do without. In our book, that's a pretty good definition of a 'bad' food.

Stripped down to basics, what the 'balanced diet' lobby is actually saying is: 'It's okay to eat bad foods as long as you also eat good foods.' What nonsense!

The so-called 'balanced diet' is really trying to persuade us to disbelieve our own trustworthy instincts about food. It is trying to convince us that eating almost *any* kind of food, no matter how unwholesome, is acceptable provided it is 'balanced' by the consumption of some magical antidote food later on. There is no scientific evidence that this 'magical antidote' theory of healthy eating is anything other than a rather cruel fairy tale.

Whenever you see an advertisement which uses those crafty words 'as part of a balanced diet', it's a strong warning that the food being given the hard sell is unhealthy. Don't swallow it!

Good Foods Make Good Diets

The French statesman General de Gaulle once remarked: 'There are three certain ways to go to hell. The first is gambling, which is the quickest. The second is women, which is the most enjoyable. The third is believing experts, which is the most certain.'

He'd obviously been listening to the views of the latest diet guru, for there are thousands, perhaps millions, of experts in the field of diet and health. Switch on your television, and you'll see them selling books, dispensing advice, plugging their products, or advising viewers. We ourselves undertake a considerable amount of lecturing and public speaking. At one health show a few years ago we were waiting behind the scenes along with several other speakers, each one selling a product or a book. A corpulent American health writer lumbered over to us with the book he'd written. 'How many have ya sold?' he demanded. We looked at each other and told him we didn't know. 'Ha!' he snorted. 'I've already sold half a million. Beat that!' His book, which seemed to promise eternal life in return for swallowing a particular type of food supplement every day, didn't square with its author – one of the most grossly overweight and hopelessly unfit men we've ever seen. A couple of years later we found out that the food supplement he was touting could actually be dangerous. By then, of course, he'd retired on his profits.

It's tragically ironic that there are so many dietary experts around and yet millions of us still die every year from diet-related diseases. Actually, this excess of experts only adds to the general confusion about healthy eating. Here's why:

- Science evolves through a dynamic process. One scientist proposes a theory; another scientist criticises it. Yet another scientist weaves the elements together to make a new theory – and so the process continues. But whose voice should you listen to?

- You know, and we know, that some experts can be bought. If you look hard enough, you can find an expert to tell you almost anything you want to hear. For example, if you happen to manufacture the world's most unwholesome junk food and you want to find an expert to tell people that it's healthier than mother's milk, then you'll eventually find one, provided you're prepared to pay . . .

- The media's job is to bring us the latest news. And that's what it generally does. But when this week's diet fad turns into next week's diet nightmare, we don't always learn about it. The next craze is already upon us.

- Ultimately, all that most experts do is to state their opinion. Which may be right, wrong – or a bit of both. Opinions are cheap; everyone's got a whole bunch, and most of us are only too eager to give them away to anyone who'll listen. Opinions are also 'pre-digested', by which we mean that they don't supply you with the knowledge or the understanding you need to form your own views. Fundamentally, most experts are really saying, 'take my word for it'. Why should we?

Thankfully, there's an easy way out of this predicament. We first proposed it in our 1992 book *Superliving!*, which was an enormous compendium of information and resources designed to give readers access to the many tools, techniques and therapies available for personal health and happiness. Its premise is simply this: 'Be your own expert'. Our philosophy in writing a book, or giving a talk, is to convey important and timely information to our readers and listeners as clearly as possible, and then to let them make their own decisions. We think this is a much more

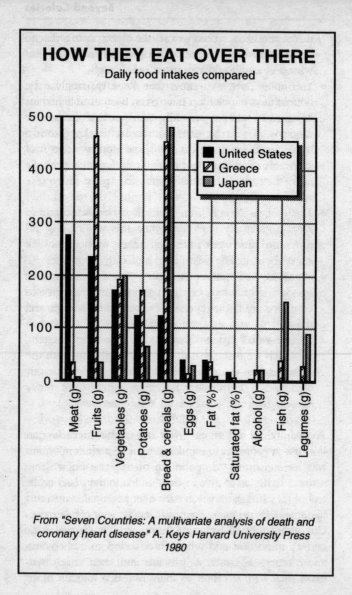

HOW THEY EAT OVER THERE
Daily food intakes compared

Legend:
- United States
- Greece
- Japan

Categories (x-axis): Meat (g), Fruits (g), Vegetables (g), Potatoes (g), Bread & cereals (g), Eggs (g), Fat (%), Saturated fat (%), Alcohol (g), Fish (g), Legumes (g)

From "Seven Countries: A multivariate analysis of death and coronary heart disease" A. Keys Harvard University Press 1980 ethical – and empowering – way of working than trying to peddle the latest food craze or diet supplement. It respects our readers and it allows us to sleep at night.

Becoming your own expert can be surprisingly easy. The basic facts of a subject have often been established for many decades and are generally undisputed. For example, you may be amazed to learn that researchers have known for decades that feeding a diet high in meat to a naturally vegetarian species, such as the rabbit, will quickly provoke heart disease. And it has also been known for an equally long time that it is virtually impossible to produce clogging of the arteries in a naturally carnivorous species (such as the dog), even when large amounts of cholesterol and saturated fat are fed to them. Elementary realities such as these can often be overlooked by today's scientists and researchers, focusing as they do upon the minutiae of scientific work. For the rest of us, however, they give us important clues to the type of natural diet which might suit us best.

In our search for 'the perfect diet', the most powerful tool of all is a relatively new science called epidemiology. As the name suggests, it evolved from the scientific study of epidemics. In 1854 a scientist called John Snow investigated and described an epidemic of cholera in London, which – by careful scientific detective-work – he found had originated from one contaminated water well. He is generally recognised as the first epidemiologist of the modern era. Now the most important point about Snow's work, and about most epidemiology, is this: he traced the cholera outbreak back to contaminated drinking water *many years before* the bacillus that causes cholera was discovered and identified. More recently, epidemiological studies have resulted in detailed descriptions of hepatitis, Lassa fever, Legionnaires' disease and toxic shock syndrome way in advance of their causative agents being identified. Also, the connection between smoking and lung cancer was first made from epidemiological studies – again, well before laboratory experiments established the cause-and-effect relationship. As epidemiology concentrates on studying the way things actually work in the real world, rather than the way laboratory scientists might like them to be, it is capable of giving us remarkably early warning signals.

Epidemiology can tell us a lot about good diets and bad diets, good foods and bad foods. When you look at all the different dietary customs, fashions, tastes and habits of the world's population, you discover some surprising things. Take a look at the chart on page 30, which compares the diets of three very different countries: the United States (a typical Western diet), Greece (a typical Mediterranean diet) and Japan (a typical Far Eastern diet). You can see that in almost every area the three countries have quite different dietary tastes. For example, meat consumption is very high in the USA, with saturated fat constituting 18 per cent of all calories consumed. Meat consumption is low in the other two countries, with saturated fat constituting 8 per cent of calorie intake in Greece and a mere 3 per cent in Japan. One of the greatest strengths of epidemiology lies in its ability to observe how diets change over time (for example, both red meat and saturated fat consumption are currently increasing rapidly in both Greece and Japan) and to relate these shifts to the changing patterns of disease and causes of death. This is one clear and straightforward way in which we can learn about the good or bad effects of the food we eat – watch what people eat and then see what they die from.

This kind of research lies at the very heart of the LifePoints system. It's not based on abstract theory. It's not trying to sell you the latest fad diet or trendy (but unproven) food supplement. It is, quite simply, utilising the priceless results obtained from the longest-running, most far-reaching experiment ever conducted in the history of the world. From North Pole to South, Far East to West, humans consume the most dramatically varying diets of any species on the face of the planet. Some of the foods we consume allow us to grow old slowly, with great vigour and vitality. Other foods seem to bestow little more than ill-health and an early grave. We know enough now to begin to put this hard-won information to practical use. And that's what *LifePoints* does.

LIFEPOINTS AND RISKPOINTS – HOW THEY WORK

If you want to start using the LifePoints system right away, turn to page 69, read the simple instructions and you'll be up and running in a couple of minutes. If you'd like to understand more about how the system works, read on.

Do you ever feel baffled when you read about the latest diet and health discoveries, such as:

- Alfalfa lowers cholesterol.
- Celery lowers blood pressure.
- Kudzu root can cure alcoholism.
- Garlic's antioxidants can fight cancer.
- Avocados lower cholesterol (yes, really).
- Phenols in red wine prevent heart disease.
- Flavonoids in fruit can prevent heart disease.
- Genistein in soya products blocks tumour growth.
- Chinese bitter melon can fight viruses, including HIV.
- Broccoli fights breast cancer by boosting anti-cancer enzymes.

News stories on all these subjects, and many similar ones, continually appear in our media. In each case, there is credible scientific evidence to support the claim being made. But, realistically, how can you actually *use* these news items? Should you try to eat a diet based on alfalfa, broccoli, celery, garlic and red wine? Doesn't that sound rather, well . . . eccentric?

And that's the problem. If you try to plan a healthy diet using nothing but scraps of information like these, you'll certainly fail – and probably go half-crazy in the process. The truth is that stories such as these have very little practical use. Yes, they're interesting to read about, but can you put the information to good use? No!

LifePoints takes exactly the opposite approach. We're interested first and foremost in the big picture. Drawing on decades of human population studies, we've built up a clear picture of the major healthy and unhealthy factors in the human diet. For example, the evidence is clear and certain that people who consume significant quantities of saturated fat have a high incidence of heart disease, so saturated fat is clearly a major risk factor in our diets. On the other hand, people who eat foods that are high in the antioxidant beta-carotene have much less heart disease and fewer cancers, which indicates that beta-carotene is one of the important health protectors. Many of these nutritional factors will already be familiar to you (all of them are described in the following section). However, never before have you had the opportunity to see how they all add up to make a healthy or unhealthy food. Now, you can.

How LifePoints Work

The task of producing LifePoint numbers for each of the foods in this book began with a truly gigantic computational effort. Over the course of several months, computers performed countless millions of calculations . . . day after day, night after night. Machines in both Europe and

America, connected through the ubiquitous Internet, facilitated our effort. Sometimes it seems that computers only serve to make our lives needlessly complicated. Yet without the awesome number-crunching power of today's computers this book could never have been possible. Gradually, the raw data began to take shape. For the first time, we began to see patterns emerging, and surprises too. Foods that we had always believed to be 'healthy' sometimes proved to be anything but. And frequently, we found ourselves bestowing a new, healthy respect on modest foodstuffs which we'd hitherto overlooked. We're certain you will share these experiences as you become familiar with the LifePoints system. Indeed, we hope you share the thrill we first felt when you realise just how effective and uncomplicated it is to use. Sheer power over your diet . . . at your fingertips!

What do LifePoints actually measure? People sometimes expect the system to be measured in calories or some other familiar unit, and are puzzled when it isn't. Well, think about it like this. Instead of measuring just one nutrient, *LifePoints* measures lots of them. First, we calculate an overall nutritional profile for the food being analysed, in its most common serving size. Next, we use a proprietary computer algorithm to compare the nutritional profile of that food to its respective 'ideal' nutritional profile, and see how it fits. A good fit earns lots of LifePoints – a bad one earns none. It is important to emphasise that we're not just adding up all the nutrients in the food. That would produce a misleading result, since foods which contain very large amounts of just one or two nutrients would come out far too favourably. A food which has a high LifePoints number provides you with *lots* of nutrients in *beneficial* amounts. And if that food is low in RiskPoints, then it's a good food. Simple, isn't it? These two numbers – LifePoints and RiskPoints – instantly provide you with a dynamic and enlightening picture of any food you care to look up!

Now let's briefly describe the importance of the nutrients we've included in the LifePoints system.

Beta-carotene   The plant form of vitamin A, beta-carotene functions as a powerful antioxidant and free radical quencher in the human body. The evidence is overwhelming that it is one of the most important nutritional factors in your armoury against ill-health. Popularly, beta-carotene is sometimes known as a 'cancer killer'. Men who eat very little beta-carotene have been shown to be seven times more likely to contract lung cancer than men whose diets are rich in it. In women, beta-carotene seems to be able to thwart cervical cancer. Further, epidemiological evidence indicates that it can also reduce the incidence of cancers of the larynx, bladder, oesophagus, stomach, colorectum and prostate gland.

Today we hear a great deal about antioxidants and free radicals in the media. The LifePoints system delivers you a diet which is naturally high in many of the most powerful antioxidants (we'll explain why taking antioxidants in their natural form is important in a moment). First, let's describe what they are. In recent years, scientists have begun to appreciate just how crucial antioxidants are to our health.

In the popular media, free radicals are often characterised as 'bad', but as in so many things, this is only partly true. The 'free radical theory' was first proposed as long ago as 1954 by Dr Denham Harman, latterly professor of medicine and biochemistry at the University of Nebraska. He discovered that radiation caused accelerated ageing and also created an excess of free radicals in body cells. What is a free radical? Simply, an atom or molecule with an unpaired electron. It is inherently unstable, as it continually searches for another molecule to which to attach itself. Gerontologist Alex Comfort wittily compared a free radical to a convention delegate away from his wife. He called it 'a highly reactive chemical agent that will combine with anything that's around'. Free radicals trigger a chain reaction that 'rusts' the body. They can damage cell membranes, proteins, carbohydrates and deoxyribonucleic acid (DNA), the genetic material of the cell and of life itself. Up to now, some sixty diseases have been associated with free radical activity, including Alzheimer's, heart disease, arthritis, multiple sclerosis and eye cataracts. Even 'liver spots' – areas of brown skin which appear on your hands and arms later in life – are connected to free radical activity. Although the body naturally produces free radicals, other substances such as cigarette smoke, radiation, air pollution, herbicides, artificial flavourings, chlorine, rancid fats, alcohol and toxic heavy metals are also causes of free radical formation.

Free radicals aren't, however, all bad. There is persuasive evidence that the basic chemicals of life first originated in the 'primeval soup' from a series of free radical reactions triggered by ionising radiation from the sun. This would explain why free radical reactions are so pervasive in nature. They enable genetic mutations to occur, and so play a pivotal role in the process of evolution. In fact, your body *deliberately* produces free radicals as part of its immune and inflammatory responses when it wants to kill invading organisms. Obviously, your body needs a system to manage free radicals effectively, and in particular there has to be an effective protective and scavenging system to ensure that they don't get out of control. That's what antioxidants do.

Beta-carotene is a natural antioxidant found in plants which is turned into vitamin A in the wall of the small intestine during digestion. Of the several hundred naturally occurring carotenoids, the most widespread and most active form is beta-carotene. Unlike vitamin A, foods which contain beta-carotene can be consumed in plentiful amounts without fear of toxicity. It is also:

- Essential for good eyesight.
- Vital for tissue growth and bone development.
- Used to maintain the integrity of mucous membranes, thus building a barrier against infection.
- Necessary for the proper growth and functioning of the reproductive system.

Taking beta-carotene, and indeed all nutrients, in their natural form is very important. In nature, nothing works in isolation. This was dramatically underlined recently, when the results of a long-awaited study came to the startling conclusion that high doses of beta-carotene, when taken in capsule form, may actually *raise* the risk of cancer rather than lower it. The first indication that a foodstuff may possess health-promoting properties frequently comes from epidemiological studies on human populations. Scientists usually react to this sort of information by trying to isolate the exact chemical or substance in the food which confers this benefit. At the end of the process is, all too often, the quest for yet another pill. As the headlines put it: 'Hopes are high that researchers may someday find dread cancers could be avoided simply by taking a daily pill . . .'

But strange and unexpected things happen when you extract one nutrient in isolation. The most recent study was intended to show whether beta-carotene protects smokers from lung cancer. Instead, it found that those taking the isolated vitamin increased their lung cancer risk by 18 per cent. The ten-year, $43 million study was conducted on 29,133 male cigarette smokers who lived in Finland. Smokers were chosen because they are already at high risk of lung cancer, and beta-carotene appeared to be especially promising as a way to lower the chance of this disease. At this stage, no one can say for sure why the researchers found this effect, but don't let's misunderstand this. This single study does *not* suggest that foods which naturally supply a plentiful amount of beta-carotene may increase your risk of cancer. Quite the opposite. Decades of studies tracking the health of thousands of people prove the wisdom of eating beta-carotene-rich foods. But whether it's wise to replace this sort of food with a pill . . . well, that's anyone's guess. What we can repeat, however, is that no nutrient works in isolation in nature. The LifePoints system gives you a way of assessing the broad nutritional profile of many different kinds of foods. It's a holistic approach – and the healthiest.

Vitamin C Long considered as relevant only to the prevention of scurvy, there is now abundant evidence that a first-class intake of vitamin C can help to prevent a wide range of human diseases. Humans are one of the few species unable to synthesise vitamin C internally, so we need to be certain of a regular, high-quality dietary intake. Vitamin C is also a very effective antioxidant and free radical quencher. You can even see it at work for yourself. Cut an apple in half and put one half aside. Pour lemon juice, which is high in vitamin C, on the other half. The half without the lemon juice will go brown through oxidation much faster than the half which is protected by the antioxidant vitamin C.

In a recent study conducted at the University of California at Berkeley, scientists isolated plasma from human blood, incubated it at body temperature and added a chemical that is known to produce free radicals as it decomposes. When vitamin C was added, it neutralised 100 per cent of the free radicals generated. Vitamin C also:

- Assists in the production of collagen, a protein which is the body's building block for all connective tissue, cartilage, bones, teeth, skin and tendons.
- Helps heal wounds, fractures, bruises and haemorrhages.
- Maintains the function of the immune system.
- Greatly facilitates the absorption of iron from the diet.
- Assists haemoglobin and red blood cell production.
- Is an essential cofactor for metabolism of many other nutrients.
- Helps the body cope with physiological and psychological stress.

Furthermore, vitamin C seems to block the formation of nitrosamines. Nitrates and nitrites are added to foods to give colour, flavour and to act as preservatives (E249–E252). During digestion these substances are converted by the human body into nitrosamines, which are known to be powerful cancer-causing chemicals (they are particularly associated with cancers of the stomach and oesophagus). The good news is that if a vitamin C-rich food is taken at the same time as foods containing nitrates or nitrites, the production of nitrosamines is greatly reduced. It has also been found that women with abnormal cervical smear results often have low amounts of vitamin C in their body. This may shed new light on the underlying damage caused by smoking because it has long been established that women who smoke have higher levels of cervical cancer. Smoking impairs the absorption of vitamin C but also requires a higher intake of vitamin C to minimise the effects of it as a pollutant.

Thiamin   Also called thiamine or vitamin B1, this was discovered to be the nutritional factor responsible for preventing the disease beriberi (Singhalese for 'I cannot', meaning that the sufferer is too ill to do anything). Epidemics of beriberi were produced in Asia by eating a diet of white polished rice, where all the nutritious outer layers of rice are discarded during processing. Although beriberi is primarily a disease of tropical countries, nutritional deficiencies of thiamin are also seen in the West, especially among people who eat a highly refined junk food diet. In the body, thiamin functions to:

- Convert carbohydrates into energy for muscles and the nervous system.
- Keep mucous membranes healthy.
- Maintain a positive mental state and possibly assist learning capacity.

Riboflavin   Also known as vitamin B2, riboflavin was first observed in 1879 as a greenish fluorescent pigment present in milk, but its function was not fully understood until 1932. It is often found in combination with other B-group vitamins, and since it is not stored in the human body for any period of time, it is vital that your diet supplies regular amounts. A deficiency will result in cracked and scaly skin, sore lips, mouth and tongue, and sometimes heightened sensitivity to light, watering of the eyes, or conjunctivitis. In the body, riboflavin works:

- With other vitamins and enzymes in using the energy from food.
- To keep mucous membranes healthy.
- As a key component in normal tissue respiration.

Niacin   Also called vitamin B3, niacin is the collective name for nicotinamide (niacinamide) and nicotinic acid. Its importance was realised in 1937 when it was discovered that the disease pellagra was caused by niacin deficiency. Lack of niacin in the diet can also lead to fatigue and muscle weakness, loss of appetite and mental unbalance. In the body, it plays an important role in:

- The release of energy from carbohydrates, fats and proteins.
- DNA synthesis.
- Keeping the skin, nerves and digestive systems working healthily.

Vitamin B6   Also known as pyridoxine, vitamin B6 is (in common with other B-group vitamins) soluble in water. This means that the body's storage capacity for B6 is limited, and we need to ensure a good daily dietary intake. It works in the body to:

- Manufacture and convert amino acids and metabolise protein.
- Produce haemoglobin.
- Convert the amino acid tryptophan to niacin.
- Facilitate the release of glycogen for energy from the liver and muscles.
- Help the body process linoleic acid (an essential fatty acid).
- Help build and maintain the integrity of the nervous system and brain.

Vitamin B12   Also called cobalamin, this vitamin is manufactured by micro-organisms such as yeasts, bacteria, moulds and some algae. The human body can store this vitamin for considerable periods (five or six years), so a daily dietary source is therefore not essential. In addition, the healthy body recycles this vitamin very effectively, recovering it from bile and other intestinal secretions, which is why the dietary requirement is so low (being measured in millionths of a gram). However, B12 deficiency is an occasional problem for people on restricted diets, and in view of its importance, it is wise to consume a known B12 food source from time to time. Its functions in the body are to:

- Facilitate the normal metabolic function of all cells.
- Work with folate to prevent anaemia.
- Assist in the synthesis of DNA.
- Promote the growth and normal functioning of the nervous system.

Folate   Folate and folacin (sometimes called vitamin B9) are the names used to describe a group of substances which are chemically similar to folic acid. Its importance to growth and the prevention of anaemia were established in 1946. The name 'folate' comes from the Latin word *folium*, meaning 'leaf', which should tell us something about the best sources of this vitamin. In the body it:

- Plays an essential role in the formation of DNA and RNA.
- Functions together with vitamin B12 in amino acid synthesis.
- Is essential for the formation of red and white blood cells.
- Contributes to the formation of haem, the iron constituent of haemoglobin.

Calcium   The most plentiful mineral in the human body, calcium amounts to 1 kilogram or so of the average adult's weight. Some 99 per cent is deposited in the bones and teeth, with the remainder fulfilling essential regulatory functions in the blood and cellular fluids. The body stores its skeletal calcium in two ways: in the non-exchangeable pool (calcium which is on 'long-term deposit' in the bones) and in the exchangeable pool, which can act as a short-term buffer to smooth over the peaks and troughs in day-to-day calcium intake. If dietary intake is consistently too low, the exchangeable pool of calcium will become so depleted that the calcium on 'long-term deposit' in the bones will be put to use, thus inducing bone degeneration.

Although calcium is often thought of as the 'bone mineral', the 1 per cent of serum calcium in the human body (calcium held outside the skeletal structure) is responsible for a vital and complex range of tasks. Calcium is clearly a critical nutrient and we all need to ensure that we have an intake. Many people erroneously believe that the consumption of heroic quantities of dairy produce is the only way to prevent bone-depleting afflictions such as osteoporosis. This is not so: the landmark China Study (as described below) showed that the Chinese eat no dairy products and take in only half the amount of calcium that Westerners do, yet osteoporosis is rare in China. Why should this be? Well, most Chinese get their calcium from vegetables. This is why we've included the calcium content of all foods in the LifePoints equation. We'd like you to get a good calcium intake from a wide variety of foods, rather than assuming that large amounts of dairy products will protect you. In fact, studies among Western vegetarians and meat-eaters show that people who eat meat and dairy products are significantly more at risk of bone loss than non-meat eaters. Calcium also helps the body to:

- Build and maintain bones and teeth.
- Control transport of chemicals across cell membranes.

- Facilitate the release of neurotransmitters at synapses.
- Influence the function of protein hormones and enzymes.
- Regulate heartbeat and muscle tone.
- Initiate blood clotting.

Iron We all know that iron prevents anaemia and is essential for haemoglobin production. As such, it is involved in the transport of oxygen from the lungs to the body's tissues, it transports and stores oxygen in the muscles, and is involved in the proper functioning of the immune system and intellect. Iron deficiency is the most common of all deficiency diseases in both developing and developed countries. Scientists vary in their estimate of what precisely constitutes a state of 'iron depletion', but the general cut-off point is variously calculated to lie between 12 and 25 micrograms of ferritin (one of the chief iron storage forms) per litre of plasma. In Britain a recent survey showed that 34 per cent of all women had a ferritin level which was under 25mcg/l and 16 per cent had less than 13mcg/l. Among men, only 6 per cent had a value of less than 25mcg/l and 3 per cent less than 13mcg/l.

These figures reflect the fact that iron is well conserved by the body (90 per cent of the 3 to 5 grams in our bodies is continually recycled). The major cause of iron depletion is loss of blood itself, as in menstruation, which on average causes about half a milligram of iron to be lost for every day of the period. However, this can vary very widely (losses as high as 1.4mg a day have been reported), so the official recommended daily allowances for women attempt to take this into account by building in a generous 'safety margin'. For example, an iron intake of 10.8mg a day appears to meet the needs of 86 per cent of all menstruating women, yet the official recommended daily allowance in the USA has been set at 15mg a day in an attempt to meet the needs of the remaining 14 per cent. This is, in fact, an uneasy compromise because even at this level of iron consumption, 5 per cent of women who have very heavy periods will not have an adequate intake to replace losses. At this point, officials either suggest that women with higher blood losses appear to compensate with an increased rate of iron absorption from their diets (USA) or 'the most practical way of meeting their high iron requirements would be to take iron supplements' (Britain). This well illustrates the dilemma facing officials whose task it is to set uniform nutritional intakes for a population whose individual needs vary very widely indeed.

The rate of absorption of iron from the diet can be significantly affected, for better or worse, by several factors. First, the rate of iron absorption is controlled by the degree to which iron is actually *needed* by the body. Normally, only 5 to 15 per cent of the iron in food is actually absorbed, but this can rise to 50 per cent in cases of iron deficiency. Second, foods containing vitamin C will considerably increase iron absorption. Iron must be delivered in a soluble form to the small intestine if it is to be absorbed, and vitamin C can make sure that non-haem iron (the sort found in plant foods) remains soluble in the acidic environment normally found there. Other organic acids found in fruit and vegetables, such as malic acid and citric acid, are also thought to possess this iron-enhancing attribute. This effect is substantial: adding 60mg of vitamin C to a meal of rice has been shown to more than triple the absorption of iron; adding the same amount to a meal of corn enhances absorption fivefold. The LifePoints formula includes both iron and vitamin C. The third factor is the tannin in tea, which can significantly reduce the absorption of iron by combining with it to form insoluble iron compounds. The food preservative EDTA can also exercise the same inhibitory effect. Both of these factors can reduce assimilation by as much as 50 per cent.

Zinc   The human body contains a mere 2 grams of zinc, distributed in the tissues in varying concentrations. Its importance to good human nutrition has only been recognised in recent years (the first reports appeared in 1963). Low zinc status manifests itself in several ways: senses of taste and smell are often decreased, wounds take longer to heal and children fail to grow properly. This is because, in the human body, zinc is:

- An essential component of many enzymes which work with red blood cells to transport carbon dioxide from tissues to lungs.
- A vital factor in many key life processes, such as our immune function and the expression of genetic information.

In addition to all the key nutrients mentioned above, the LifePoints number assesses foods for their protein content and also for their fibre content, which as you must know, imparts a whole host of health benefits, ranging from the prevention of various forms of cancer to lowering blood cholesterol and preventing constipation. A high LifePoints number indicates that the food concerned is a plentiful source of the nutrients mentioned above. A low number indicates that it is a poor source.

When you consider that the LifePoints system rates foods for all the nutrients just mentioned and ensures that you don't consume dangerous levels of the unhealthy ingredients, you can see why we say that LifePoints is 'beyond calories'.

How Riskpoints Work

There is one unequivocal risk factor in the diets most of us eat today, and that is the amount of fat consumed. Fat — particularly saturated fat (mainly from animal sources) – is without doubt our number one dietary enemy. Most of us already know that eating too much fatty food is supposed to be bad for us. But we'll bet you didn't know the following shocking and startling facts:

- Eating 100 calories from fat will make you put on more weight than eating 100 calories from carbohydrate. On the face of it, it seems impossible – after all, 100 calories is 100 calories no matter where it comes from – right? Wrong! Your body stores surplus energy intake in the form of fat. When you eat fatty foods, your body can very easily and very efficiently turn that food fat into body fat; only about 3 per cent of the fat you consume is burnt up by your body in the storage process. Building massive hips and thighs has never been easier! However, the process of turning carbohydrate-rich foods into body fat consumes a considerable proportion (about 25 per cent) of their calories. Furthermore, carbohydrate-rich meals boost your body's metabolism, which in turn makes it harder for you to gain weight. Fatty foods simply don't work this way.
- If you want to control your weight, all types of fat are equally bad. Forget the advertising slogans about polyunsaturates and monounsaturates . . . none of them help you shed those pounds. One gram of fat, of any kind, yields twice as many calories as a gram of protein or a gram of carbohydrate. Fat is a poor nutritional return on your food investment.
- A naturally low-fat diet can do remarkable things, including reverse heart disease. Scientifically, there's

no remaining doubt. The plaques which build up and eventually block coronary arteries can be unblocked by eating a good, low-fat diet. Among other benefits, an increased flow of blood in these arteries can also reduce the pain of angina.

One simple RiskPoints number manages to achieve two important goals with regard to fat. Firstly, it ensures that your total fat consumption remains healthily low. How low? Well, if your RiskPoints daily total adds up to no more than 100, you'll have eaten no more than 40 grams of fat. For the average woman, whose energy intake comes to about 2,200 calories, that represents 16 per cent of calories. For a man, consuming about 2,900 calories, it keeps your total fat intake down to about 12 per cent of calories. These are the kinds of levels which research shows our species has naturally consumed for most of our history. In many parts of the world – China, for example – people still consume this (to us) relatively low level of fat in their diets. The result? Many of the 'diseases of civilisation' which so plague us in the West are virtually unknown. Why do we suggest you keep your fat intake down to this level? Here's how the *New York Times* put it when reporting the results of the largest ever scientific study into the diets and health of the Chinese people: 'Reducing dietary fat to less than 30 per cent of calories, as is currently recommended for Americans, may not be enough to curb the risk of heart disease and cancer. To make a significant impact, the Chinese data imply, a maximum of 20 per cent of calories from fat – and preferably only 10 to 15 per cent – should be consumed.'

The China Study is a turning point in the science of epidemiology. The study began in 1983, with the aim of exploring the dietary causes of cancer. Since then, it has been expanded to include heart, metabolic and infectious diseases. And these findings are only the beginning. Dr T. Colin Campbell, a nutritional biochemist from Cornell University who masterminded the study, predicts that this 'living laboratory' will continue to generate vital findings for the next forty to fifty years. Already, the China Study has confirmed that obesity is clearly related to *what* you eat, rather than how much. The Chinese actually consume 20 per cent *more* calories than Westerners do, but Westerners are 25 per cent fatter. The culprit? All that fat in our food.

Keep your RiskPoints to about 100, and you'll be eating a naturally low-fat diet. But that's by no means all it does for you. The RiskPoints number also intelligently guides you away from food which is unhealthily high in saturated fat, and steers you towards food which is low in it. Why is this important? Because saturated fat is clearly linked to the development of coronary heart disease, and probably to certain cancers, too. In this respect, all fat is not the same. We don't want you getting all your fat intake as unhealthy saturated fat, so the RiskPoints formula penalises foods which are too high in this type of fat. You can think of this part of the RiskPoints equation as a silent friend there in the background, gently nudging you away from unhealthy foods and leading you to the healthier choices. You may not notice it, but it's there, working for you all the time.

Just imagine what would happen if all the world were to eat a natural diet which was high in LifePoints and low in RiskPoints. Actually, we don't have to imagine. The science of epidemiology already suggests what many of the benefits could be:

- Bolstering the immune system.
- Preventing coronary heart disease.

- Reversing coronary heart disease.
- Preventing cancers.
- Delaying the ageing process.
- Preventing cataracts.
- Preventing osteoporosis.
- Preventing and treating high blood pressure.
- Preventing strokes.
- Preventing impotence.
- Preventing and treating obesity.
- Treating arthritis.
- Preventing gout.
- Preventing and treating diabetes.
- Preventing hypoglycaemia.
- Preventing and treating constipation.
- Preventing varicose veins.
- Preventing appendicitis.
- Preventing gallstones.
- Reducing food poisoning.

Sounds like a pretty healthy world, doesn't it?

PART 2
ANSWERS TO ALL YOUR QUESTIONS

We've found that when people start using the LifePoints system, the same sorts of questions crop up again and again. Here they are . . . together with the answers.

Do I have to make allowances for the freshness of food?

Food quality is a very important issue to us. The level of nutrition you receive from your diet depends not only on what food you choose to eat, but also – among other things – on how you store and cook it. This provides at least three opportunities for nutrient loss. If you lead a hectic, demanding life, you need these nutrients even more and therefore need to know how you can safeguard them. Unfortunately, we can't know how fresh, or otherwise, the food is you buy. So please read and take to heart the advice that follows.

Choosing food
- The more a foodstuff is processed, the greater the loss of natural nutrients, so buy only unprocessed wholefoods.
- If possible, buy organic food, preferably from local producers. Organic foods are more likely to have their nutrients intact and, if they are from local producers, they will not have been in lengthy storage during transit. Nutrients decay with time, so eat close to the soil. Also, the risk of pesticide residue is remote.

Pesticides are poisons – their basic purpose is to kill. In an ideal world, pesticides are not supposed to leave any residue on food by the time it's ready to eat, but considerable evidence indicates that food *can* be tainted with pesticide residue, even if it's been washed many times. Farmers spend twice as much on herbicides as they do on insecticides and fungicides put together. Herbicides are used to kill off weeds either by preventing their growth or sometimes by causing unnaturally rapid growth. Many are designed to be absorbed directly into the system of the plant itself, so it is impossible to get rid of them simply by washing. One such systemic herbicide was 2,4,5-T (short for 2,4,5-trichlorophenoxy acetic acid), which was an ingredient in Agent Orange, the chemical used by the US Army in Vietnam to destroy the food supply of the Vietcong and to strip them of cover in areas of dense vegetation. At the time it was first used, there was no evidence that Agent Orange might be harmful, but years later the effects started to be noticed. Vietnamese exposed to it showed an unusually high level of clinical abnormalities, such as miscarriages, birth defects and sterility. American soldiers also became ill, with ailments ranging from cancer to deformations in their children. The probable cause of these devastating problems was another substance present in the herbicide called dioxin, which is formed during the 2,4,5-T manufacturing process. Exposure to dioxin can disrupt the body's white blood cells and so reduce its ability to fight off disease.

Another connection between the use of herbicides and human illness was revealed when a scientist exposed a statistical connection between the use of herbicides and Parkinson's Disease, which affects the central nervous system. It is suspected that a certain group of herbicides (chemically very similar to MPTP, a designer drug known to produce an irreversible Parkinsonian-like syndrome in humans) is capable of bringing about the slow destruction of a specific group of brain cells, thus causing Parkinson's Disease. Again, this effect can take many years to happen, making it very difficult for scientists to prove that there's a health problem – until it's too late.

Thankfully, many supermarket chains have now started to stock organic produce. So what is organic food? The Soil Association states that, 'Organic food is produced responsibly, taking account of the needs of consumers, farm animals and the environment. Organic farmers produce food which:

Is grown without artificial pesticides and fertilisers.
Tastes good rather than just looks good.
Is never irradiated.
Contains no artificial hormones, genetically manipulated organisms or unnecessary medication.
Is not over-processed to remove the goodness.
Does not contain flavourings, dyes and other additives.
Is nutritious, living food which promotes positive health and well-being.'

Organic food is also better for the environment. Intensive agriculture is responsible for about 50 per cent of all water pollution (such as high nitrate levels). It has been clearly established that modern biological-organic farming methods lead both to lower leaching of nitrates into the water supply and to lower nitrate content in vegetables.

If you can't afford to eat organic food all the time (and it *can* be very expensive), at least try to make sure that your children eat as organically as possible. Children are much more vulnerable than adults to the toxic effects of chemical residue. 'Children's systems can retain a greater portion of a given toxin because their gastrointestinal tract is more easily penetrated,' says Dr Steven Markowitz, assistant professor in the division of environmental and occupational medicine at Mount Sinai School of Medicine in New York City. 'And kids eat more per unit weight than adults do, so the tissues in their bodies may be more exposed to these substances.' On top of this, children are dramatically more susceptible to carcinogens than adults are because infancy and childhood are periods of rapid cell division. 'The cells of many different tissues in the body are proliferating, and that increases the chances that a genetic change leading to cancer will result,' says Markowitz. So if you can't afford to provide organic food for all the family, do try giving it to just the youngest – they are the most at risk from the long-term health effects of pesticides.

- Check the use-by date. Old produce will have suffered severe nutritional decay. Shopkeepers always put older stock at the front of the display, so buy from the back.
- Canning and bottling processes reduce the levels of vitamin C, thiamin and folic acid. Vitamin C loss continues during storage. If you have to buy canned food, use it as soon as possible.
- Avoid foods that contain sulphur dioxide as a preservative – they will have almost entirely lost their thiamin (vitamin B1) content.
- Freeze-dried foods are relatively good since there is no heating to deplete nutrients.
- Frozen foods suffer some thiamin and vitamin C loss. However, the loss is less than in fresh food which has been kept for a number of days. If shopping for fresh food is a problem for you, frozen foods are probably the next best alternative, but be careful not to overcook them (see below).

- Choose unrefined monounsaturated oils – preferably olive oil – for cooking. Pure, refined polyunsaturated oils turn rancid more easily.
- Don't buy damaged tinned goods, no matter how good a bargain they appear to be. Small cracks in the lining of the cans affect the contents, which will certainly affect the delicate vitamins and other nutrients, and may even cause the food itself to turn bad.

Storage

- Store oils, fats and oily foods like cheeses and shelled nuts in the refrigerator. This will help to slow down the process of oxidation which turns them rancid.
- Vitamin C, thiamin, riboflavin and folic acid all decay quickly in air. Once vegetables are harvested, the damaged tissues release an enzyme that starts to destroy the vitamin C. Blanching inhibits the enzyme, which is why freezing fresh vegetables is much better than keeping them unfrozen and eating them many days later.
- Vegetables lose around 70 per cent of their folic acid content within three days if they are stored in daylight. Store vegetables in the refrigerator until you are ready to use them, or freeze them straight away.
- Store grains and cereals whole and in a dry, cool place.

Cooking

- Cooking is generally harmful to the nutrients in food. However, it also changes starches, proteins and some vitamins into accessible forms for us, as well as releasing nutrients in some foods which are otherwise bound in, like the amino acid tryptophan in cornmeal. Cooking is necessary for other foods to destroy toxic substances such as those found in soybeans and kidney beans. Cooking also makes some foods, like meat, palatable to eat. However, there are ways in which you can reduce the nutrient loss in foods during the cooking process.

- Pressure cooking is perhaps the best way to reduce nutrient loss. Invest in a non-aluminium pressure cooker which, because of the reduced cooking bills, will also reduce energy consumption and therefore the size of your fuel bills.

- After pressure cooking, the next healthiest options are steaming and microwaving. Steamers are also a lot cheaper to buy than a microwave oven. Further down the list are boiling, grilling, stir frying (at high temperature where the fat seals in the nutrients), sautéing and deep frying.

- If you cook with fat, don't let it become so hot that it starts to smoke. At this temperature the essential fatty acid linoleic acid is destroyed immediately.

- Fats which have been used for cooking once must be discarded since the linoleic acid and vitamins A and C will have been lost.

- If you boil food, do so for the minimum amount of time and then use the water for stock afterwards. The fragile water-soluble vitamins, as well as some minerals, leach into cooking water, which is why soups are so nutritious.

- Don't add bicarbonate of soda to cooking water, even if your cookbook recommends it; it destroys valuable B vitamins.

- Prepare food immediately before cooking as vitamin C is destroyed once cells are damaged in vegetables; for the same reason, try not to chop them too finely. Scrubbing vegetables is better than peeling them.

- Once prepared, steam or cook the vegetables in boiling water straight away.

- Use pans with close-fitting lids and avoid using copper pans, which encourage oxidation and vitamin C loss.

- Once food is cooked, eat it straight away. Keeping it warm will only result in further nutrient loss, which is why eating out too frequently may be less than healthy for you.

If you lead a hectic lifestyle and consider that you don't have time for some of the advice given above, think again. The life you lead is totally dependent on a good nutritional support system, without which you're running on empty. And you can only do that for so long. Shopping regularly for fresh foods can appear to present a problem if you don't attach a high priority to it. But just think – no sensible person buys a Rolls-Royce, then tries to run it on two-star petrol. It's the same with your body – the better the fuel, the better the performance you'll receive.

Do I have to follow the measurements given?

The more accurate you can be with your measurements, the better the system will work for you. To make things as easy as possible, most of the foods are listed in common measurements (a cup, a slice and so on). Remember, we want you to eat as widely as possible. Do you know what the prime cause of malnutrition is? Most people in the West often erroneously believe that it's lack of food, but that's not true. The principal cause of malnutrition is lack of variety of food. A monotonous diet is a dangerous diet. To encourage you to choose as widely as possible, we suggest:

- If you want to eat *less* than the stated serving size, simply divide the LifePoints and RiskPoints appropriately (e.g. if you eat half the serving size, simply divide them by two).
- If you want to eat *more* than the stated serving size, multiply the RiskPoints appropriately (e.g. if you eat

twice the serving size, multiply the RiskPoints by two) but the LifePoints stay unchanged.

How accurate are the numbers?

As accurate as we can make them. In practice, this means that we've used food values collected from the world's leading authorities for our calculations. The major variable is, inevitably, the quality and freshness of the food concerned (see above). However, let's also realise that men and women don't live by numbers alone. At the end of the day the most important function the LifePoints and RiskPoints figures serve is to awaken in you your own instinctive sense of a healthy diet. We don't want you to be a slave to the numbers – we want you to use them to educate and liberate.

Can't I just subtract the RiskPoints from the LifePoints to produce one simple number?

No. When we were first developing the system, we tried very hard to achieve this. But because they are essentially two completely different measures of a food's worth, it is not possible to combine them meaningfully. However, we think having two numbers is actually superior to having one. This is why: one number tells you very little about the good and bad ingredients in a foodstuff. It doesn't allow you to make a mental picture of that food, nor does it allow you to see how and where that food might fit into your diet. Having two index numbers allows you to get more of a *feel* for the food concerned, which is what we want. When you've used the system for a day or two, you'll see what we mean.

What happens if I exceed my daily RiskPoints?

In all probability, you won't drop dead. However, it's a strong indication that you're not eating the healthiest diet you could. Just try gradually to get these RiskPoints down to 100 or so. It may take some time to re-educate your tastebuds, particularly if you're used to a high-fat diet, but don't feel dejected if you can't hit the 100 mark instantly. The LifePoints system is a tool; use it as you would any other to achieve your success over a period of time.

If I hit 100 daily LifePoints, does it guarantee that I've got all my recommended daily allowances?

Recommended daily allowances (RDAs), like calories, are dangerous things. One of the most dangerous things they do is to give people a false sense of security that they're well nourished. RDAs are, in reality, best guesses by a panel of government officials. When the US Department of Agriculture released its 'dietary pyramid', this is what the eminent nutritional authority Walter C. Willett, of the Harvard School of Public Health, had to say about it in *Science* magazine: 'Inevitably, such a document represents a mix of well-supported findings, educated guesses, and political compromises with powerful economic interests such as the dairy and meat industries.'

Another hopeless problem with RDAs is that they're entirely impossible for ordinary people to use. Just adding up your daily food intake for one nutrient is difficult enough, but when you have to cope with a dozen or more, and watch your fat, and calories, and endlessly juggle your daily menu to make sure you hit all your RDAs . . . forget it! Ultimately, trying to follow any RDA system leads to one thing only (apart, that is, from madness). Pills – that's the only way you can guarantee that you're getting 100 per cent of the recommended daily intake for specific vitamins and minerals. And as we've already seen (under beta-carotene), pills are not a substitute for a healthy diet.

We don't want you to hit 100 LifePoints and then sit back. See if you can get it higher – write to us, and tell us how high. The RDA approach implies that a certain (guestimated) level of nutrition is all you need to bother with. Increasingly, this assumption is being challenged and discredited as old science. The LifePoints system goes way beyond RDAs. By showing you the good, high-nutrient foods and steering you away from the empty or hazardous foods, you're getting the big picture. Eating a high-quality diet is far more important than worrying whether your vitamin C consumption is 55 grams or 60 grams. And that's what LifePoints can do for you.

How can I put together meals and recipes using LifePoints?

Easily. Remember to go for variety. Choose from all of the first four groups. When you've chosen a food from one group, go to another for your next food choice. As far as recipes are concerned, we'd like you to try *The LifePoints Cookbook*, which shows you just how easy it is to produce delicious food using the system. And it gives you over 150 quick, easy and economical recipes, too.

I eat out a lot; how can I cope in restaurants?

The same way you'd cope at home or in the supermarket. Use LifePoints to help you choose good food. Beware sauces, dressings and other easily overlooked 'invisible' foods. You'll find them all listed here, so there's no excuse to forget them.

I've heard that plants contain natural chemicals which cause cancer, so nothing's really safe to eat, is it?

Yes, some plants certainly do produce chemicals to defend themselves against fungi, insects and animal predators. Consider the cabbage. It contains forty-nine natural pesticides and metabolites, many of which may be cancer-causing or cancer-promoting. Actually, it's been estimated that there are between 5,000 and 10,000 natural pesticides and associated breakdown products in our diets. And we eat about 1.5 grams of them every day. But wait! Before you decide to give up eating for good, consider this. Even though people who eat cabbages are certainly taking in all those natural pesticides which the cabbage uses to defend itself, those same people actually have a greatly reduced risk of getting cancer. Further, research shows that cabbage may actually retard existing cancers from spreading (metastasis). So what's going on? Simply this. *Nothing works in isolation.* A naturally healthy diet contains more than enough life-protecting nutrients and other factors to block the effect of minor plant toxins. So don't give up on the cabbage.

What about alcohol?
Thanks, we'll have two small glasses of red wine, please.

No, where does alcohol fit into the system?
It doesn't. Basically, our advice is to restrict your alcohol consumption to the occasional glass of red wine. In most countries, high dietary intakes of saturated fats are strongly associated with high coronary heart disease death rates. Some regions of France, however, are an important exception to this rule; they have low death rates from heart disease despite high-fat diets. This paradox is almost certainly due to the antioxidant phenolic compounds contained in red wine (and as we all know, the French *do* drink red wine). No other alcohol has this effect.

Why are meat, fish and dairy products an optional group?
Simply because research shows that people who don't eat these products are generally healthier than those who do.

63

I'm not just fat, I'm flabby. What can I do about that?

Skin is elastic and after a time it will tighten up. But you can help it and your muscles by doing regular exercise. Join a local keep fit or yoga class to use all your muscles in a gentle and gradual stretching programme. Your muscles will change shape as a result and you will regain some of the curves and corners you used to be so proud of. Alternatively, take up walking as your form of fitness training. Brisk, determined walking is actually an aerobic exercise that helps you lose weight, improve respiration and increase your stamina. Start with a minimum of thirty minutes per day, four times per week. Remember, keep the pace brisk and slightly challenging – you should feel slightly breathless, but always able to talk as you walk.

I'm really very overweight and I don't fancy joining an exercise class. I know that exercise helps to reduce weight, but I don't know what exercise to take in my condition.

The LifePoints system can help you to lose weight by retraining your tastebuds. In addition, you could try walking (as above), or you might purchase one of the many audio or video cassettes on the market that are aimed at stretching only. (Do not try one of the aerobic programmes at this point.) Or, if you have a staircase in your home, you could practise stepping. Simply step up one step, then step down again – 100 times at a speed that will enable you to continue talking. Do not become breathless; if you do, slow down. Swimming is also a very beneficial exercise which you can do by yourself. It is an excellent means of improving your overall muscle tone.

I really go to pieces at Christmas and other special occasions.

High days and holidays are full of family and social

pressures and the appeal of traditional foods. *The Life-Points Cookbook* has plenty of ideas for you to consider for celebrations and entertaining. We think food should be fun.

What should I do when I feel weak-willed and want to eat something with a high RiskPoints number?

Choose something else. There are plenty of foods with respectable LifePoints numbers and zero or little Risk-points. Remember – you're in control. You eat what you want to eat. The LifePoints system is all about taking charge of your own diet. If you want to choose bad food, then that's your decision – we're not going to nag you. But here's a tip: immediately you sense that feeling, take out a notepad and write down exactly what you want to eat, and put its RiskPoints number beside it in BIG NUMBERS. Now look at what you've written. Your inclination to eat that thing is guaranteed to diminish.

I always start diets but then get fed up cooking two meals – one for myself and another for my family.

This is a difficult problem, but not an impossible one. First, sit down with your family and tell them about the LifePoints system. Then tell them that it is difficult to make two meals and that this has, in the past, caused you many problems with diets. Your family is certain to come up with a number of ideas that will help. They may even decide they want to eat healthily, too!

I have always been a fast eater. When I finish my first serving, my family isn't even halfway through theirs, so I usually take another serving just to keep them company. I know this has caused a lot of my weight problems, but how can I slow down?

There are a number of simple, unobtrusive little techniques you can use to help you eat more slowly.

- Don't cut your food into pieces all at once (if it needs cutting). Instead, cut one bite-sized piece at a time, eat it, then cut the next piece.
- Take a forkful of food, then put your fork down on the side of your plate while you chew that mouthful. Don't pick up the next forkful until you have swallowed the first.
- Buy a set of pretty cloth napkins and use one at each meal. Wipe your mouth frequently during the meal to help slow you down.
- Take a slow, deep breath in and out between each mouthful of food. This will take the hurry out of eating and also keep you relaxed.
- With all this slow eating, you might think your food will go cold. Warm your plate before serving to prevent this. Also, take small portions of food so that the rest remains in the hot serving dish.

I use a lot of oil and fat in cooking and I've got used to the flavour. What is a good substitute for all this fat?

Cut the fat in cooking to an absolute minimum. Ignore the fat included in the recipes you use, but, when it seems essential, try cutting the amount listed in half. You could also try the following tips.

- Blend a little tomato or tandoori paste with 2 fl oz (60ml) water and pour into your pan. Place over a high heat and when the liquid bubbles, add your vegetables and stir frequently. This is what we call the 'new sauté' method; the liquid replaces the fat normally used in a sauté. You will be surprised at how tasty this is.
- Try *The LifePoints Cookbook*.

I have a really sweet tooth that always gets the better of me. What can I do to stop myself eating sweet things?

There's nothing at all wrong in eating sweet foods such as fresh fruit: use LifePoints to find the best. But as far as puddings and desserts are concerned, a sweet tooth is really a bully that always wants to have its own way. You will have to turn it gradually into a more respectable creature. Start by depriving your sweet tooth, a little at a time, of what it wants. Instead of a chocolate bar, eat some dried figs or raisins. Instead of sugary tea or coffee, drink it unsugared with a piece of sugarless oat cake to give you slow-release energy. Next, try retraining your sweet tooth to become a sour tooth. The flavours are equally strong, but the effects are wonderfully different. Every time you want a sweet 'injection', chew on a wedge of lemon, take a sip of cider vinegar in water, or eat a gherkin. Finally, give yourself time to break the sweet habit. If you have one or two bad days, don't give up. Keep going and you will succeed.

PART 3
PUTTING LIFEPOINTS TO WORK

––––––

If you can count to 100, you can use LifePoints. Let's show you how, then we'll answer some of the common questions people often have.

All the foods that follow have been carefully and painstakingly analysed to reveal their overall nutritional profile. Each food has two numbers:

The LifePoints number is a measure of the food's healthy components – the higher the number, the healthier the food.

The RiskPoints number is a measure of the food's unhealthy components – the higher the number, the more unhealthy the food.

A food with high RiskPoints and no LifePoints is a 'bad' food. Similarly, a food with high LifePoints and no RiskPoints is a 'good' food. Your aim is to maximise the number of LifePoints you consume and minimise the RiskPoints. How many RiskPoints and LifePoints should you consume? It's simple:

Your LifePoints should total at least 100 per day.

> **Your RiskPoints should total no more than 100 per day.**

That's all the adding up you have to do. Now you know the way the LifePoints system works. It's much easier than calorie counting because you don't have to add up to 1,000 or more. And, uniquely, the LifePoints system gives you a feeling for the food itself. Use it for just a day or two and you'll find that your instincts for good food and bad food are revived and developed. That's why we say LifePoints is an empowering system.

LifePoints Guidelines

1. For your convenience, the foods are divided into six major groups, and there's a comprehensive index at the back as well. To eat a healthy and varied diet, you must choose foods from the first four groups.

Groups 5 and 6 are optional. The suggested number of servings per day from each group is listed below:

Group 1	Fruit and Fruit Juices	3 servings
Group 2	Cereals, Grains and Pasta	4 servings
Group 3	Vegetables and Vegetable Products	4 servings

Group 4	Legumes, Nuts and Seeds	3 servings
Group 5	Meat, Fish and Dairy Products	optional
Group 6	Drinks, Desserts, Snacks and Sauces	optional

2. Variety is the keynote of healthy eating, so to encourage you to eat as wide a variety as possible, please observe the following rule:

> The LifePoints for any foodstuff can be counted only once no matter how often you eat that food during the day. This means that if you eat the same food twice, only its RiskPoints count for the second helping. In other words, don't try to cheat the system by eating ten servings of broccoli for 120 LifePoints and only 10 RiskPoints. (If you ever did eat ten helpings of broccoli, using this simple rule you'd accumulate 10 RiskPoints but only 12 LifePoints.)

3. Foods are listed in common serving sizes, but it's quite acceptable to halve or even quarter the servings provided you also reduce the associated RiskPoints and LifePoints.

People are not always used to sitting down and planning their day's diet. Too often our food consumption is the last thing we think about, when it should really be the first – and sometimes it's not easy to decide where to begin. Well, now it is easy.

PLANNING YOUR DAY'S DIET

Let's follow a tradition and plan a day's diet by thinking in terms of breakfast, lunch, dinner and perhaps a mid-morning and mid-afternoon snack. First, we'll plan a day's meals without referring to the *LifePoints* list, and outline a menu that is familiar after years of use. Perhaps you could follow our example and outline one of your own at the same time. Here's ours:

BREAKFAST

Food	RiskPoints	LifePoints
1/2 grapefruit	0	2
2 slices wholewheat bread toasted	6	3
with 2 pats butter	36	0
and 2 tablespoons jam	0	0
1 cup black coffee	0	0

LUNCH

Food	RiskPoints	LifePoints
Baked potato filled with sour cream and chives	56	16
Mixed side salad	0	9
1 tablespoon thousand island dressing	13	0
1 can carbonated soft drink	0	0

DINNER

Food	RiskPoints	LifePoints
1 fillet baked sole	4	18
Scalloped potatoes	50	12
Boiled peas	0	9

Apple crumble	21	3
1 cup black coffee	0	0

SNACKS

Food	RiskPoints	LifePoints
2 cups tea with milk, no sugar	24	3
2 digestive biscuits	2	0
1 slice fruit cake	9	1

After you've outlined your day's diet, look each food up in the listing of over 1,500 foods in this book. If you can't find a food at first, use the comprehensive index to learn its page number: you will soon become familiar with how the foods are grouped. As you find each food, make a note of the food group in which it is listed.

Note the RiskPoints and LifePoints indicated for each food and write these beside the foods in your list – as we've illustrated in our day plan. Note that we've followed the rule (given under point 2 of LifePoints Guidelines) which asks you to count only the Risk-Points of second or third helpings of the same food. So in our menu, we've two servings each of toast, coffee, tea and digestive biscuits. For each of them, we've doubled the RiskPoints but counted LifePoints for only one serving.

When you have dealt with each food in your day's diet, add up how many different foods you have chosen from each of the six *LifePoints* food groups. For instance, in the menu we have listed above, the foods are allocated in the following way:

Fruit and Fruit Juices	1 serving
Cereals, Grains and Pasta	1 serving
Vegetables and	4 servings

Vegetable Products	
Legumes, Nuts and Seeds	0 servings
Meat, Fish and Dairy Products	2 servings
Drinks, Desserts, Snacks and Sauces	8 servings

Next, add up the total number of RiskPoints and write that number at the bottom of the menu. Now add up the total number of LifePoints and write that number at the bottom too. In the diet we've outlined, the totals are:

RiskPoints	221
LifePoints	76

That's it. You have a *LifePoints* profile of your day's diet. What does it tell you?

Well, in a nutshell, we could do better. For a start, we do not have great variety in our diet, as indicated by the allocation to food groups given above: we are worryingly short of foods from Fruits and Fruit Juices; Cereals, Grains and Pasta; and Legumes, Nuts and Seeds. Foods in those groups provide so much that is essential to long-term good health that a lifetime of menus such as this one will almost guarantee illness and early demise. In addition, we have a very large selection of foods from Drinks, Desserts, Snacks and Sauces, an optional food group because there is not much in that group to bring good health yet plenty that will undermine it. The good news is that we have met the LifePoints recommendations for variety in the Vegetables and Vegetable Products food group by selecting four different foods. This is excellent and we will build on this feature when we amend the day's diet.

Just a quick word, before we rework the menu, about

the total points we achieved. The RiskPoints total is more than double its recommended maximum, while the Life-Points total is far too low. This is a fatty, over-processed, low-nutrient diet.

Now let's see if we can improve it. Start with breakfast again. It's not a bad breakfast, except that it's too sweet and fatty. Let's keep it similar but reduce the fat and replace the jam with a fresh fruit instead:

BREAKFAST

Food	RiskPoints	LifePoints
1/2 grapefruit	0	2
1/2 cantaloupe melon	1	10
2 slices wholewheat bread, toasted	6	3
with 2 teaspoons yeast extract	0	11
1 cup black coffee	0	0

The lunch had two servings of vegetables, so we'll keep those, but it was treacherously high in fat. Let's drop the sour cream and find something else to put on the potato. No, not butter. We're short of legumes, so how about baked beans? The salad is nice, but can we reduce the fattiness of the dressing? We don't need the fizzy drink either, but we do enjoy a slightly sweet drink so . . .

LUNCH

Food	RiskPoints	LifePoints
Baked potato	0	12
topped with ½ cup/126g baked beans	1	8
Mixed side salad	0	9

1 tablespoon low-fat thousand island dressing	4	0
1 cup/8 fl oz fresh orange juice	1	9

Dinner sounded delicious and filling, didn't it? Again, it was a bit fatty and over-processed. Let's start from scratch with this meal.

DINNER

Food	RiskPoints	LifePoints
Gazpacho soup	5	5
1 wholewheat roll	3	3
Mixed side salad	0	9
1 tablespoon low-fat French dressing	2	0
Lasagne made with TVP mince	25	43
3 matzo crackers	0	3
with bean pâté	0	11
1 cup black coffee	0	0

Finally, let's see if we can lift the snacks out of the doldrums.

SNACK ONE

Food	RiskPoints	LifePoints
Milkshake made from 1 fresh banana	1	6
and 1 cup soya milk	11	7

SNACK TWO

Food	RiskPoints	LifePoints
1 glass/6 fl oz carrot juice	0	13

1 apple	1	1

Now let's analyse this day's diet. The foods can be allocated as follows:

Fruit and Fruit Juices	5 servings
Cereals, Grains and Pasta	4 servings
Vegetables and Vegetable Products	6 servings
Legumes, Nuts and Seeds	3 servings
Meat, Fish and Dairy Products	0 servings
Drinks, Desserts, Snacks and Sauces	3 servings

So far, very good. Now the RiskPoints and LifePoints.

RiskPoints	61
LifePoints	165

Wonderful! With not too much adjustment we have turned a fatty, over-processed diet into a low-fat, high-nutrient diet. In fact, the RiskPoints are low enough that we could, for instance, spread margarine as well as yeast extract on our toast, and use a standard rather than low-fat salad dressing. And as you can see, this day's diet is not restrictive: one wouldn't feel hungry or deprived. Yet this day's diet provides the variety and nutritional value that can help ensure you are providing a healthy diet for you and your family; one that will improve and build their health for the future. Try it. You will notice positive health effects within a few days.

SUPERCHARGING THE SYSTEM

The LifePoints system is very flexible, and can be customised to suit your individual requirements. Here are some suggestions:

- Although we suggest initially setting a maximum RiskPoints total of no more than 100 per day, this limit can be reduced if needed. For example, for a potent cholesterol-lowering regime, you might choose to observe a limit of 50 RiskPoints daily (this would ensure you consumed no more than 20 grams of fat in your diet, only a small proportion of which would be saturated). People respond very individually to diet therapy, so a little experimentation and fine tuning might be necessary. Obviously, you should also seek the advice of your medical or health specialist in formulating an effective therapy.

- Don't make the mistake of thinking that 'zero-zero' foods can be eaten abundantly. People who are used to counting calories occasionally confuse the Life-Points system with their previous dietary regime. It's not the same at all! Foods which have no RiskPoints and no LifePoints ('zero-zero') are empty foods, and have little place in your diet strategy. Remember, you have two objectives: 1) to achieve a high LifePoints score and 2) to keep your RiskPoints within the designated limit. Zero-zero foods do *not* help you to achieve your prime dietary goal of a healthy LifePoints score. Eating a zero-zero food is counter-productive, because it makes it less likely that you'll have room or the appetite to eat higher-scoring foods during the day. The LifePoints system helps you prioritise your food intake. Zero-zero foods are very low priority.

- Don't feel guilty about your fragmented eating habits. Today, most of us don't have the opportunity to sit down to three square meals a day . . . we snack when we can, and maybe eat only one 'proper' meal a day. Sociologists call this 'grazing', and in some respects it mirrors our primate ancestors' feeding habits. Strangely, most food and recipe books blindly fail to recognise that this is how most people actually eat (for one book that's ideal for grazers, read the companion volume to this work, *The LifePoints Cookbook*). The LifePoints system is perfectly attuned to this modern way of eating because it focuses on your total daily food intake. The one danger of grazing is simply that you consciously or subconsciously eat sub-optimal food, telling yourself that you'll 'eat a good meal later'. LifePoints can help you here, showing you how to choose the best snacks to eat. So stop feeling ashamed of your snacking, and instead, see it positively – as a new way of achieving positive nutrition with the help of the LifePoints system.
- Be aware that certain groups of the population have enhanced nutritional needs. In today's society, where food is so plentiful, it may seem strange to think that under-nutrition can occur at all, but the evidence shows that it can. Although you can substantially increase your overall nutrient intake by following the LifePoints system, you should still be aware that some nutrients are not particularly easy to obtain from day-to-day food sources.

Calcium   If your dietary intake of this vital mineral is consistently too low then bone degeneration may occur. Many people incorrectly suppose that the consumption of copious amounts of dairy produce is the only way to prevent bone-depleting afflictions such as osteoporosis. This isn't true – strangely enough, people who eat meat and dairy products are significantly more at risk of bone loss than non-meat eaters. Good plant food sources of calcium include blackstrap molasses, sesame seeds, tofu, green leafy vegetables such as collards, cabbage, almonds and carob flour. Calcium is best absorbed when you have adequate vitamin D in your body (sunlight is a good source) and when there's plenty of boron in the diet (available in apples and other fresh fruits and vegetables).

Iron   A nutrient well conserved by the body (90 per cent of the 3 to 5 grams in our bodies is continually recycled). The major cause of iron depletion is loss of blood itself – as in menstruation. Women of childbearing years should therefore take care to eat good dietary sources, which include: blackstrap molasses, pumpkin and squash seeds, spirulina, many fortified breakfast cereals, quinoa, dried mixed fruit, wheatgerm and kidney beans. Foods which contain vitamin C (e.g. fresh fruit and vegetables) will considerably increase your absorption. Several factors can significantly reduce its absorption of iron, among them tea (the tannin forms insoluble iron compounds) and the food preservative EDTA. Both of these can reduce assimilation by as much as 50 per cent.

Vitamin B12   If you are eating a diet composed exclusively of plant-based foods (i.e. from the first four groups only), then make sure you sometimes consume a good source of vitamin B12, such as fortified breakfast cereal, fortified soya milk, yeast extract or fermented food such as tempeh.

THE TOP TEN FOODS FROM EACH GROUP

People often ask us to nominate our 'top ten' foods from each of the four essential groups. Here they are, together with their associated RiskPoints and LifePoints.

GROUP ONE: FRUIT AND FRUIT JUICES

	RISKPOINTS ✗	LIFEPOINTS ✔
Papaya: fresh	1	12
Melon: cantaloupe	1	10
Orange juice: fresh	1	9
Guavas: fresh	2	9
Pineapple juice	0	8
Apricots: dehydrated	0	8
Prunes: dehydrated	1	7
Mangoes: fresh	1	7
Figs: dried	2	7
Bananas: fresh	1	6

GROUP TWO: CEREALS, GRAINS AND PASTA

	RISKPOINTS ✗	LIFEPOINTS ✔
Raisin Bran	1	32
Grape Nuts	0	23
All Bran	1	22
Semolina	2	18
Wheatgerm: toasted	7	18
Soya flour: low-fat	7	17
Cornflakes	0	16
Porridge: made with skimmed milk	5	13
Millet: cooked	6	12
Pizza: with tomatoes and olives, no cheese	8	10

GROUP THREE: VEGETABLES AND VEGETABLE PRODUCTS

	RISKPOINTS ✗	LIFEPOINTS ✔
Spinach: boiled	1	25
Baked potato topped with baked beans	1	20
Asparagus: canned	4	18
Turnip greens: boiled	0	16
Broccoli: fresh	1	14
Beansprouts: stir-fried	0	11
Yeast extract: fortified with vitamin B12	0	11
Squash: baked	3	10
Vegetables: mixed, canned	1	10
Green beans: canned	0	10

GROUP FOUR: LEGUMES, NUTS AND SEEDS

	RISKPOINTS ✗	LIFEPOINTS ✔
Textured vegetable protein (TVP)	2	21
Baked beans: on toast, no butter	4	17
Lentils: boiled	0	16
Adzuki beans: boiled	0	13
Kidney beans: boiled	1	12
Chickpeas: boiled	5	12
Bean pâté: made with lentils	0	11
Peas: split, boiled	0	9
Broad beans: boiled	0	9
Ginkgo nuts: dried	1	6

To help you plan your day's diet, photocopy the following form and carry it with you. More menu suggestions as well as individual recipes and advice on composing your own recipes are included in *The LifePoints Cookbook*.

LIFEPOINTS DAILY PLANNER

	RISKPOINTS ✗	LIFEPOINTS ✓
YOUR DAILY TOTAL:		

PART 4
FOOD GROUPS

GROUP 1 – FRUIT AND FRUIT JUICES

	RISKPOINTS ✗	LIFEPOINTS ✔
Apples: canned slices, drained (½ cup/102g) 68 cals	1	0
Apples: dehydrated (low-moisture), sulphured, stewed (½ cup/97g) 72 cals	0	0
Apples: dehydrated (low-moisture), sulphured, uncooked (½ cup/30g) 104 cals	0	1
Apples: dried, sulphured, stewed (½ cup/128g) 73 cals	0	1
Apples: dried, sulphured, uncooked (5 rings/32g) 78 cals	0	1
Apples: fresh with skin (1 fruit/138g) 81 cals	1	1
Apples: fresh without skin (1 fruit/128g) 73 cals	0	1
Apples: juice, canned or bottled, with added vitamin C (1 cup/8 fl oz/248g) 117 cals	0	3
Apples: juice, canned or bottled, without added vitamin C (1 cup/8 fl oz/248g) 117 cals	0	1
Apples: without skin, boiled (1 cup/171g) 91 cals	1	1

	RISKPOINTS ✘	LIFEPOINTS ✔
Apples: without skin, micro-waved (1 cup/170g) 95 cals	1	1
Apple sauce: canned, sweetened (½ cup/128g) 97 cals	0	1
Apple sauce: canned, un-sweetened with added vitamin C (½ cup/122g) 52 cals	0	1
Apple sauce: canned, un-sweetened without added vitamin C (½ cup/122g) 52 cals	0	1
Apricot nectar: canned, with added vitamin C (1 cup/8 fl oz/251g) 141 cals	0	4
Apricot nectar: canned, without added vitamin C (1 cup/8 fl oz/251g) 141 cals	0	3
Apricots: canned in heavy syrup, without skins, solids & liquid (1 cup/258g) 214 cals	0	4
Apricots: dehydrated (low-moisture), sulphured, stewed (½ cup/124g) 156 cals	0	6
Apricots: dehydrated (low-moisture), sulphured, uncooked (½ cup/60g) 192 cals	0	8
Apricots: dried, sulphured, stewed with added sugar (½ cup halves/135g) 153 cals	0	3

	RISKPOINTS ✗	LIFEPOINTS ✔
Apricots: dried, sulphured, stewed without added sugar (½ cup halves/125g) 106 cals	0	4
Apricots: dried, sulphured, uncooked (10 halves/35g) 83 cals	0	3
Apricots: fresh (3 fruits/106g) 51 cals	1	3
Avocado: see Vegetables and Vegetable Products group		
Bananas: dehydrated or banana powder (1 tbsp/6.2g) 21 cals	0	0
Bananas: fresh (1 fruit/114g) 105 cals	1	6
Blackberries: canned in heavy syrup, solids & liquid (½ cup/128g) 118 cals	0	4
Blackberries: fresh (1 cup/144g) 75 cals	1	6
Blackberries: frozen, unsweetened (1 cup/151g) 97 cals	1	7
Blackcurrants: fresh (½ cup/56g) 35 cals	0	2
Blueberries: canned in heavy syrup, solids & liquid (½ cup/128g) 113 cals	1	1
Blueberries: fresh (1 cup/145g) 81 cals	1	3

	RISKPOINTS ✗	LIFEPOINTS ✔
Boysenberries: canned in heavy syrup (½ cup/128g) 113 cals	0	4
Breadfruit (¼ small fruit/96g) 99 cals	0	3
Carissa (Natal plum) (1 fruit/ 20g) 12 cals	0	0
Cherries: sour red, canned, solids & liquid (½ cup/122g 44 cals	0	2
Cherries: sour red, fresh (1 cup with stones/103g) 52 cals	0	2
Cherries: sweet, canned, solids & liquid (½ cup without stones/125g) 68 cals	0	2
Cherries: sweet, fresh (1 cup/ 145g) 104 cals	3	3
Crab apples: fresh (1 cup slices with skin/110g) 84 cals	0	1
Cranberries: fresh (1 cup whole/95g) 47 cals	0	1
Cranberry: juice cocktail (1 cup/8 fl oz/253g) 144 cals	0	2
Cranberry: sauce, canned, sweetened (½ cup/138g) 208 cals	0	1
Cranberry-apple juice drink (1 cup/8 fl oz/245g) 164 cals	0	2
Currants: zante, dried (½ cup/72g) 204 cals	0	6
Custard apple: see Soursop		

	RISKPOINTS ✗	LIFEPOINTS ✔
Dates: fresh and dry (10 fruits/83g) 228 cals	0	5
Feijoa (1 fruit/50g) 25 cals	0	1
Figs: canned in heavy syrup, solids & liquid (3 fruits plus 1¾ tbsp liquid/85g) 75 cals	0	1
Figs: dried, stewed (½ cup/130g) 140 cals	1	5
Figs: dried, uncooked (5 fruits/93g) 237 cals	2	7
Figs: fresh (1 medium fruit/50g) 37 cals	0	1
Fruit salad (peach, pear, apricot, pineapple & cherry) canned in light syrup, solids & liquid (½ cup/126g) 73 cals	0	1
Fruit salad: tropical (pineapple, papaya, banana & guava) canned in heavy syrup, solids & liquid (½ cup/128g) 110 cals	0	2
Gooseberries: canned in light syrup, solids & liquid (½ cup/126g) 92 cals	0	2
Gooseberries: fresh (½ cup/75g) 33 cals	1	2
Granadilla: see Passion-fruit		
Grape juice: canned or bottled unsweetened (1 cup/8 fl oz/253g) 154 cals	0	3

	RISKPOINTS ✗	LIFEPOINTS ✔
Grapefruit: fresh (½ fruit/ 120g) 38 cals	0	2
Grapefruit juice: canned, sweetened (1 cup/8 fl oz/ 250g) 115 cals	0	4
Grapefruit juice: canned, unsweetened (1 cup/8 fl oz/ 247g) 94 cals	0	4
Grapefruit sections canned in light syrup, solids & liquid (½ cup/127g) 76 cals	0	2
Grapes: fresh (10 fruits/50g) 36 cals	0	1
Grapes: Thompson seedless, canned in heavy syrup, solids & liquid (½ cup/128g) 93 cals	0	2
Grapeseed oil: see Margarines, Oils & Spreads in the Drinks, Desserts, Snacks and Sauces group		
Guava: fresh (1 cup/165g) 84 cals	2	9
Guava sauce: cooked (½ cup/ 119g) 43 cals	0	3
Kiwifruit (Chinese gooseberries): fresh (1 medium fruit/76g) 46 cals	0	2
Kumquats: fresh (4 fruits/80g) 50 cals	0	3
Lemon juice: canned or bottled (1 cup/8 fl oz/244g) 51 cals	1	4

	RISKPOINTS ✗	LIFEPOINTS ✔
Lemon juice: canned or bottled (1 tbsp/15g) 3 cals	0	0
Lemon juice: fresh (1 cup/8 fl oz/244g) 61 cals	0	5
Lemon juice: fresh (1 tbsp/15g) 4 cals	0	0
Lemons: fresh, without peel (1 medium fruit/58g) 17 cals	0	1
Lime juice: canned or bottled, unsweetened (1 cup/8 fl oz/246g) 52 cals	1	3
Lime juice: canned or bottled, unsweetened (1 tbsp/15g) 3 cals	0	0
Lime juice: fresh (1 cup/8 fl oz/246g) 66 cals	0	3
Lime juice: fresh (1 tbsp/15g) 4 cals	0	0
Limes: fresh (1 fruit/67g) 20 cals	0	1
Lychees: fresh (1 cup/190g) 125 cals	2	4
Mangoes: fresh (1 fruit/207g) 135 cals	1	7
Melons: cantaloupe, fresh (½ fruit/267g) 93 cals	1	10
Melons: honeydew, fresh (1 cup cubed pieces/170g) 60 cals	0	3

	RISKPOINTS ✗	LIFEPOINTS ✔
Mixed fruit (peach, pear & pineapple) canned in heavy syrup, solids & liquid (½ cup/ 128g) 92 cals	0	2
Nectarines: fresh (1 fruit/ 136g) 67 cals	1	2
Orange & apricot juice drink (1 cup/8 fl oz/250g) 128 cals	0	3
Orange drink: canned (1 cup/ 8 fl oz/248g) 126 cals	0	2
Orange drink: carbonated (12 fl oz can/372g) 179 cals	0	0
Orange juice: canned, unsweetened (1 cup/8 fl oz/ 249g) 105 cals	0	7
Orange juice: fresh (1 cup/8 fl oz/248g) 112 cals	1	9
Orange juice: fresh (juice from 1 fruit/86g) 39 cals	0	3
Orange juice: made from concentrate (1 cup/8 fl oz/ 249g) 110 cals	1	7
Oranges: fresh (1 fruit/131g) 62 cals	0	6
Papayas: fresh (1 fruit/304g) 119 cals	1	12
Passion-fruit: fresh (1 fruit/ 18g) 17 cals	0	0
Passion-fruit juice: fresh (1 cup/8 fl oz/247g) 126 cals	0	5

	RISKPOINTS ✘	LIFEPOINTS ✔
Peach nectar: canned with added vitamin C (1 cup/8 fl oz/249g) 134 cals	0	2
Peach nectar: canned without added vitamin C (1 cup/8 fl oz/249g) 134 cals	0	2
Peaches: canned in heavy syrup, solids & liquid (½ cup/128g) 95 cals	0	1
Peaches: dehydrated (low-moisture), sulphured, stewed (½ cup/121g) 161 cals	1	4
Peaches: dehydrated (low-moisture), sulphured, uncooked (½ cup/58g) 189 cals	1	5
Peaches: dried, sulphured, stewed without added sugar (½ cup halves/129g) 99 cals	0	3
Peaches: dried, sulphured, uncooked (5 halves/65g) 155 cals	1	5
Peaches: fresh (1 fruit/87g) 37 cals	0	1
Pear nectar: canned with added vitamin C (1 cup/8 fl oz/250g) 150 cals	0	2
Pear nectar: canned without added vitamin C (1 cup/8 fl oz/250g) 150 cals	0	1
Pears: Asian, fresh (1 fruit/122g) 51 cals	0	1

	RISKPOINTS ✗	LIFEPOINTS ✓
Pears: canned in heavy syrup, solids & liquid (half a pear with 1¾ tbsp liquid/79g) 58 cals	0	0
Pears: dried, sulphured, stewed without added sugar (½ cup halves/128g) 163 cals	0	3
Pears: dried, sulphured, uncooked (5 halves/87g) 228 cals	1	4
Pears: fresh (1 fruit/166g) 98 cals	1	2
Persimmons: fresh (1 fruit/ 25g) 32 cals	0	0
Pineapple juice: canned, unsweetened without added vitamin C (1 cup/8 fl oz/ 250g) 140 cals	0	7
Pineapple juice: canned, unsweetened with added vitamin C (1 cup/8 fl oz/ 250g) 140 cals	0	8
Pineapple: canned in heavy syrup, solids & liquid (1 slice with 1¼ tbsp liquid/58g) 45 cals	0	1
Pineapple: canned in heavy syrup, solids & liquid (½ cup chunks or tidbits/128g) 100 cals	0	2
Pineapple: fresh (1 slice 3½ in diam./84g) 41 cals	0	2

	RISKPOINTS ✗	LIFEPOINTS ✔
Plantain: cooked (½ cup slices/77g) 89 cals	0	3
Plums: canned in heavy syrup, solids & liquid (3 fruits with 2¾ tbsp liquid/133g) 118 cals	0	2
Plums: fresh (1 fruit/66g) 36 cals	1	1
Plums: fresh (½ cup slices/83g) 46 cals	1	1
Pomegranate: fresh (1 fruit/154g) 105 cals	1	2
Pomelo (shaddock): fresh (1 fruit/609g) 231 cals	0	11
Prickly pears: fresh (1 fruit/103g) 42 cals	1	2
Prune juice: canned (1 cup/8 fl oz/256g) 182 cals	0	8
Prunes: canned in heavy syrup, solids & liquid (5 fruits with 2 tbsp liquid/86g) 90 cals)	0	3
Prunes: dehydrated (low-moisture), stewed (½ cup/140g) 158 cals	0	4
Prunes: dehydrated (low-moisture), uncooked (½ cup/66g) 224 cals	1	7
Prunes: dried, stewed without added sugar (½ cup without stones/106g) 113 cals	0	4

	RISKPOINTS ✗	LIFEPOINTS ✓
Prunes: dried, uncooked (5 fruits without stones/42g) 100 cals	0	3
Quinces: fresh (1 fruit/92g) 52 cals	0	1
Raisins: seeded (½ cup packed/82g) 243 cals	1	5
Raisins: seedless (½ cup packed/82g) 246 cals	0	5
Raspberries: canned in heavy syrup, solids & liquid (½ cup/128g) 116 cals	0	3
Raspberries: fresh (1 cup/123g) 60 cals	1	6
Raspberries: frozen (½ cup/125g) 129 cals	0	4
Redcurrants: fresh (½ cup/56g) 31 cals	0	1
Rhubarb: cooked with sugar (½ cup/120g) 139 cals	0	3
Satsuma: see Tangerines		
Soursop: fresh (½ fruit/312g) 206 cals	4	18
Starfruit: fresh (1 fruit without seeds/127g) 42 cals	1	2
Strawberries: canned in heavy syrup, solids & liquid (½ cup/127g) 117 cals	0	4
Strawberries: fresh (1 cup/149g) 45 cals	1	5

	RISKPOINTS ✗	LIFEPOINTS ✓
Sultanas (½ cup packed/82g) 248 cals	0	5
Tamarinds: fresh (1 fruit/2g) 5 cals	0	0
Tangerine juice: fresh (1 cup/ 8 fl oz/247g) 106 cals	1	4
Tangerines: canned in light syrup (½ cup/126g) 77 cals	0	2
Tangerines: fresh (1 fruit/84g) 37 cals	0	3
Watermelon: fresh (1/16 fruit/ 482g) 154 cals	5	10
Whitecurrants: fresh (½ cup/ 56g) 31 cals	0	1

GROUP 2 – CEREALS, GRAINS AND PASTA

	RISKPOINTS ✗	LIFEPOINTS ✔

Breakfast Cereals

The average weight of most servings of breakfast cereals is about one ounce (28g): first choose your cereal, then add either whole, semi-skimmed, skimmed or soya milk as below.

	RISKPOINTS ✗	LIFEPOINTS ✔
40% bran flakes (1 oz/28g) 93 cals	1	32
All Bran: wheat bran (1 oz/28g) 71cals	1	22
Cornflakes: honey and nut (1 oz/28g) 113 cals	3	16
Cornflakes: regular (1 oz/28g) 110 cals	0	16
Cornflakes: sugar frosted (1 oz/28g) 108 cals	0	16
Crispy wheat & raisins (1 oz/28g) 99 cals	1	20
Frosted rice crispies (1 oz/28g) 109 cals	0	16
Grape Nuts (1 oz/28g) 101 cals	0	23
Muesli: homemade, oats with wheatgerm & nuts (1 oz/28g) 138 cals	19	5

	RISKPOINTS ✗	LIFEPOINTS ✔
Oat flakes: fortified (1 oz/28g) 105 cals	1	27
Raisin bran (1.3 oz/36g) 115 cals	1	32
Shredded Wheat: large biscuit (2 biscuits/38g) 133 cals	1	6
Shredded Wheat: small biscuits (1 oz/28g) 102 cals	1	5
Special K: low-calorie rice & wheat (1 oz/28g) 111 cals	0	21
Sugar Smacks (1 oz/28g) 106 cals	1	16
Weetabix (2 biscuits/37.5g) 124 cals	2	9
Wheatgerm : toasted, plain (1 oz / 28g) 108 cals	7	18

	RISKPOINTS ✗	LIFEPOINTS ✔
Milk: cow's, whole (the serving for a bowl of cereal is about ¾ cup/183g) 117 cals	37	9
Milk: cow's, semi-skimmed (¾ cup/183g) 101 cals	16	10
Milk: cow's, skimmed (¾ cup/183g) 64 cals	1	9
Milk: soya (¾ cup/183g) 60 cals	8	5

	RISKPOINTS ✗	LIFEPOINTS ✔

Cooked Breakfast Foods

For egg dishes, see Eggs in the Meat, Fish and Dairy Products group.

	RISKPOINTS ✗	LIFEPOINTS ✔
Ground rice cereal: cooked with water (¾ cup/183g) 95 cals	0	1
Semolina cereal: cooked with water (¾ cup/188g) 100 cals	0	7
French toast: with butter (2 slices/135g) 356 cals	58	15
Instant oats: fortified, plain, prepared with water (1 serving/177g) 104 cals	4	25
Instant oats: fortified, with apples & cinnamon, prepared with water (1 serving/149g) 136 cals	4	23
Muffin: plain, prepared with whole milk (1 muffin/57g) 172 cals	17	6
Muffin: blueberry, prepared with whole milk (1 muffin/57g) 165 cals	16	5
Pancakes: made with blueberries (1 pancake/38g) 84 cals	8	3
Pancakes: plain (1 pancake/38g) 86 cals	9	3

	RISKPOINTS ✗	LIFEPOINTS ✔
Pancakes: with butter and syrup (3 pancakes/232g) 520 cals	43	15
Porridge made with semi-skimmed milk (¾ cup/210g) 205 cals	19	15
Porridge made with skimmed milk (¾ cup/210g) 168 cals	5	13
Porridge: made with soya milk (¾ cup/207g) 163 cals	12	10
Porridge: made with water (¾ cup/175g) 109 cals	4	4
Porridge: made with whole milk (¾ cup/210g) 221 cals	33	13
Waffles: plain (1 waffle/75g) 218 cals	26	9

Breads

There are many breads and bread products in the world, most of which are extremely delicious and very healthy, too. Here we've gathered comprehensive information for many of the most common kinds. Also, we've pre-calculated LifePoints and RiskPoints data for many popular sandwiches and burgers, so you can instantaneously compare one with another. And to make things even easier, we've even

	RISKPOINTS ✗	LIFEPOINTS ✔
calculated data for a 'basic sandwich', to which you can add any filling you choose.		
Bagels: cinnamon-raisin (3½ in bagel/71g) 195 cals	3	8
Bagels: egg (3½ in bagel/71g)	3	9
Bagels: plain or with onion, poppy or sesame seed (3½ in bagel/71g) 195 cals	2	10
Baker's yeast: compressed (1 cake/0.6 oz/17g) 18 cals	0	13
Banana bread: made with margarine (1 slice/60g) 196 cals	15	3
Banana bread: made with vegetable shortening (1 slice/60g) 203 cals	17	3
Basic sandwich: 2 slices of wholewheat bread & margarine . . . add your own filling (55g) 140 cals	10	7
Breadcrumbs: dry, grated, plain (1 oz/28g) 112 cals	3	6
Breadcrumbs: dry, grated, seasoned (1 oz/28g) 104 cals	1	3
Breadsticks: plain (1 stick/10g) 41 cals	2	1
Bread: made with oat bran (1 slice/30g) 71 cals	3	4

	RISKPOINTS ✗	LIFEPOINTS ✔
Bread: made with oatmeal (1 slice/27g) 73 cals	2	3
Brioche: *see* Egg bread		
Chapati: made without fat (1 medium/35g) 71 cals	0	2
Ciabatta: *see* Italian bread		
Cornbread: made with low-fat milk (1 piece/65g) 173 cals	11	7
Croissant: apple (57g) 145 cals	18	4
Croissant: cheese (57g) 236 cals	41	8
Croissant: chocolate (72g) 310 cals	86	8
Croissant: made with butter (57g)	50	6
Croissant: with egg, cheese and ham (152g) 474 cals	131	20
Croûtons: commercial (¼ cup/ 7g) 31 cals	1	1
Crumpet: plain, toasted (52g) 133 cals	2	6
Crumpet: with butter (63g) 189 cals	18	8
Dinner roll: *see* Wholewheat roll; White bread roll		
Dumplings (2 average/60g) 127 cals	29	2
Egg bread (brioche) (1 slice/ 40g) 115 cals	6	6

	RISKPOINTS ✗	LIFEPOINTS ✔
French bread (1 medium slice/25g) 69 cals	1	3
French roll (38g) 105 cals	4	5
Granary bread: toasted (1 slice/25g) 73 cals	2	3
Hamburger or hotdog buns (1 bun/43g) 123 cals	5	5
Irish soda bread (1 slice/60g) 174 cals	7	5
Italian bread (1 slice/30g) 81 cals	2	4
Pitta bread: white (1 pitta/60g) 165 cals	1	8
Pitta bread: wholewheat (1 pitta/64g) 170 cals	4	8
Pizza: with cheese (1 slice/⅛ of a pizza/63g) 140 cals	11	11
Pizza: with cheese, meat & vegetables (1 slice/⅛ of a pizza/79g) 184 cals	13	11
Pizza: with pepperoni (1 slice/⅛ of a pizza/71g) 181 cals	17	10
Pizza: with tomatoes & olives, no cheese (1 slice/⅛ of a pizza/63g) 142 cals	8	10
Pumpernickel (1 slice/32g) 80 cals	2	4
Raisin bread (1 slice/26g) 71 cals	2	3

	RISKPOINTS ✗	LIFEPOINTS ✔
Rye bread (1 slice/32g) 83 cals	2	4
Scones: plain or buttermilk (1 scone/35g) 127 cals	14	3
Toast: wholewheat, with butter (1 slice/30g) 105 cals	27	3
Toast: wholewheat, with margarine (1 slice/30g) 105 cals	13	3
Toast: wholewheat, with 1 tsp olive oil (1 slice/30) 113 cals	15	3
Vienna bread: see French bread		
White bread: soft (1 slice/25g) 67 cals	2	3
White bread: toasted (1 slice/23g) 67 cals	2	3
White bread: roll (1 roll/28g) 77 cals	4	3
Wholewheat bread: soft (1 slice/25g) 62 cals	2	3
Wholewheat bread: toasted (1 slice/25g) 62 cals	2	3
Wholewheat roll (28g) 75 cals	3	3
Yorkshire pudding (1 individual pudding/30g) 65 cals	10	1

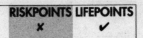

	RISKPOINTS ✗	LIFEPOINTS ✔

Sandwiches and burgers

For the following popular fillings, turn to the relevant group.

Bacon: *see* Pork in the Meat, Fish and Dairy Products group
BLT: *see* Pork in the Meat, Fish and Dairy Products group
Cheese & pickle: *see* Cheese in the Meat, Fish and Dairy Products group
Cheese & tomato: *see* Cheese in the Meat, Fish and Dairy Products group
Cheeseburgers: *see* Beef in the Meat, Fish and Dairy Products group
Chicken fillet: *see* Chicken in the Meat, Fish and Dairy Products group
Egg & cheese: *see* Eggs, chicken in the Meat, Fish and Dairy Products group
Egg mayonnaise: *see* Eggs, chicken in the Meat, Fish and Dairy Products group
Egg, cress & mayonnaise: *see* Eggs, chicken in the Meat, Fish and Dairy Products group

	RISKPOINTS ✗	LIFEPOINTS ✔
Ham & cheese: *see* Pork in the Meat, Fish and Dairy Products group		
Ham, egg & cheese: *see* Pork in the Meat, Fish and Dairy Products group		
Hamburgers: *see* Beef in the Meat, Fish and Dairy Products group		
Luncheon meat sandwich: *see* Pork in the Meat, Fish and Dairy Products group		
Peanut butter & banana: *see* Nuts in the Legumes, Nuts and Seeds group		
Peanut butter & jam: *see* Nuts in the Legumes, Nuts and Seeds group		
Pork & beef paste: *see* Pork in the Meat, Fish and Dairy Products group		
Roast beef: *see* Beef in the Meat, Fish and Dairy Products group		
Roast beef with cheese: *see* Beef in the Meat, Fish and Dairy Products group		
Sandwich spread: *see* the Vegetables and Vegetable Products group		
Steak sandwich: *see* Beef in the Meat, Fish and Dairy Products group		

	RISKPOINTS ✘	LIFEPOINTS ✔
Tuna salad: *see* Fish & Seafood in the Meat, Fish and Dairy Products group		
Vegetable burger: *see* Legume & Bean Products in the Legumes, Nuts and Seeds group		

Crackers

For sweet biscuits, see Biscuits & Cookies in the Drinks, Desserts, Snacks and Sauces group

	RISKPOINTS	LIFEPOINTS
Crackers: standard snack-type (4 crackers/14g) 71 cals	10	1
Cream crackers (1 cracker/ 3g) 13 cals	0	0
Crispbread: rye (1 slice/10g) 37 cals	0	1
Matzos (1 matzo/28g) 112 cals	0	3
Melba toast (1 slice/5g) 20 cals	0	0
Oatcakes (1 biscuit/10g) 44 cals	4	1
Rice cakes: made with brown rice (1 cake/9g) 35 cals	0	1
Rice cakes: made with brown rice and buckwheat (1 cake/ 9g) 34 cals	0	1
Rice cakes: made with brown rice and corn (1 cake/9g) 35 cals	0	0

	RISKPOINTS ✗	LIFEPOINTS ✓
Rice cakes: made with brown rice and sesame seed (1 cake/9g) 35 cals	0	1
Rice cakes: made with brown rice, multigrain (1 cake/9g) 35 cals	0	1
Rusks (1 rusk/10g) 41 cals	1	1
Taco shells: baked (1 medium/13g) 61 cals	7	1
Tortillas: ready-to-bake or fry (1 medium/25g) 56 cals	1	2
Water biscuits: see Matzos		

Grains and Flours

	RISKPOINTS ✗	LIFEPOINTS ✓
Amaranth: boiled (½ cup/ 66g) 14 cals	0	6
Arrowroot flour (⅓ cup/43g) 154 cals	0	0
Barley: pearled cooked (1 cup/157g) 193 cals	1	8
Buckwheat flour: whole-groat (½ cup/60g) 201 cals	4	12
Buckwheat groats: roasted cooked (1 cup/198g) 182 cals	3	6
Bulgur: cooked (1 cup/182g) 151 cals	1	8
Corn bran: crude (⅓ cup/ 25g) 56 cals	0	5
Cornflour (1 tbsp/8g) 30 cals	0	0

	RISKPOINTS ✗	LIFEPOINTS ✔
Cornmeal (polenta): wholegrain yellow (½ cup/61g) 221 cals	5	8
Couscous: cooked (1 cup/179g) 200 cals	0	6
Couscous: prepared with chickpeas & mixed vegetables (1 cup/179g) 208 cals	16	8
Millet: cooked (1 cup/240g) 286 cals	6	12
Oat bran: cooked (½ cup/110g) 44 cals	2	3
Oats (½ cup/78g) 303 cals	13	14
Popcorn: see Snacks & Sweets in the Drinks, Desserts, Snacks and Sauces group		
Quinoa (1 cup/170g) 636 cals	24	32
Rice bran: crude (⅓ cup/28g) 88 cals	14	22
Rice: brown, long-grain, cooked (1 cup/195g) 216 cals	4	7
Rice: brown, medium-grain, cooked (1 cup/195g) 218 cals	4	6
Rice flour: white (½ cup/79g) 289 cals	2	5
Rice: white, glutinous, cooked (1 cup/241g) 234 cals	1	3

	RISKPOINTS ✗	LIFEPOINTS ✓
Rice: white, long-grain, cooked (1 cup/158g) 205 cals	1	6
Rice: white, long-grain, parboiled & cooked (1 cup/175g) 200 cals	1	7
Rice: white, long-grain, precooked or instant (1 cup/165g) 162 cals	0	4
Rice: white, medium-grain or Italian, cooked (1 cup/186g) 242 cals	0	7
Rice: white, short-grain or pudding, cooked (1 cup/186g) 242 cals	0	7
Rye flour: medium dark (½ cup/51g) 181 cals	2	6
Semolina (½ cup/84g) 302 cals	2	18
Soya flour: low-fat (½ cup stirred/44g) 143 cals	7	17
Wheat bran: crude (2 tbsp/7g) 15 cals	0	3
Wheatgerm oil: see Margarines, Oils & Spreads in the Drinks, Desserts, Snacks and Sauces group		
Wheatgerm: crude (¼ cup/29g) 104 cals	7	16
White wheat flour: plain (½ cup/62g) 226 cals	1	11

	RISKPOINTS ✗	LIFEPOINTS ✔
White wheat flour: self-raising, enriched (½ cup/62g) 219 cals	1	12
Wholewheat flour: wholegrain (½ cup/60g) 203 cals	2	11
Wholewheat: sprouted (⅓ cup/36g) 71 cals	1	3
Wild rice: cooked (½ cup/ 82g) 83 cals	0	4

Pasta

Note: the cooked pasta listed below is plain-boiled unless stated otherwise.

	RISKPOINTS ✗	LIFEPOINTS ✔
Cannelloni: meat-filled (3 tubes/300g) 334 cals	42	23
Lasagne: made with mince (1 serving/1 cup/300g) 458 cals	75	34
Lasagne: made with TVP mince (1 serving/1 cup/300g) 351 cals	25	43
Macaroni: baked with cheese (1 serving/1 cup/200g) 348 cals	74	12
Macaroni: durum wheat, eggless, cooked (1 cup/140g) 197 cals	2	7
Macaroni: wholewheat, eggless, cooked (1 cup/140g) 174 cals	1	6

	RISKPOINTS ✗	LIFEPOINTS ✓
Noodles: Chinese, cooked (1 cup/45g) 237 cals	34	7
Noodles: egg, cooked (1 cup/160g) 213 cals	5	9
Noodles: egg with spinach, cooked (1 cup/160g) 211 cals	6	12
Noodles: Japanese, soba, cooked (1 cup/114g) 113 cals	0	3
Noodles, Japanese, somen, cooked (1 cup/176g) 231 cals	0	2
Pasta & bean soup (1 cup/8 fl oz/253g) 195 cals	12	10
Pasta: all shapes, egg, cooked (1 cup/140g) 182 cals	6	8
Pasta: all shapes, eggless, cooked (1 cup/140g) 183 cals	3	7
Pasta: spinach, cooked (1 cup/140g) 182 cals	3	9
Ravioli: with spinach and cheese filling (1 serving/1 cup/240g) 308 cals	41	21
Risotto: alla Milanese, with meat (1 serving/1½ cups/225g) 240 cals	35	16
Risotto: alla Piemontese, vegetarian with parmesan cheese (1 serving/1 cup/150g) 209 cals	36	6

	RISKPOINTS ✗	LIFEPOINTS ✔
Spaghetti: bolognese (1 serving/2 cups/410g) 538 cals	57	31
Spaghetti: in four cheeses sauce (1 serving/2 cups/449g) 1106 cals	384	41
Spaghetti: plain, cooked (1 cup/140g) 197 cals	2	7
Spaghetti: wholewheat, cooked (1 cup/140g) 174 cals	1	6
Spaghetti: with Italian sauce – tomatoes, mushrooms, ham, olive oil (1 serving/2 cups/382g) 466 cals	49	18
Spaghetti: with pesto sauce (1 serving/1 cup/255g) 429 cals	43	16
Spaghetti: with simple tomato sauce, made from tomatoes, onion, garlic, olive oil and green pepper (1 serving/2 cups/322g) 303 cals	27	12

GROUP 3 – VEGETABLES AND VEGETABLE PRODUCTS

	RISKPOINTS ✗	LIFEPOINTS ✔
Alfalfa seeds: sprouted (1 cup/33g) 10 cals	0	2
Artichokes (globe or French): boiled (½ cup hearts/84g) 42 cals	0	5
Asparagus: boiled (½ cup/ 90g) 22 cals	0	10
Asparagus: canned, drained solids (1 can/248g) 47 cals	4	18
Asparagus: soup, cream of (1 cup/8 fl oz/244g) 85 cals	10	4
Aubergine: boiled (½ cup 1 in cubes/48g) 13 cals	0	1
Aubergine: fried in olive oil (½ cup cubes/63g) 137 cals	35	1
Avocado: dip (guacamole) (½ cup/138g) 184 cals	40	11
Avocado: fresh (½ fruit/100g) 161 cals	38	9
Avocado: vinaigrette (½ fruit with 1 tbsp dressing) 231 cals	57	9
Bamboo shoots: boiled (1 cup ½ in slices/120g) 14 cals	0	2
Bamboo shoots: stir-fried in light oil (1 cup/125g) 59 cals	13	2
Batavia: see Chicory greens		

	RISKPOINTS ✗	LIFEPOINTS ✔
Beansprouts: mung, fresh (1 cup/104g) 31 cals	0	7
Beansprouts: mung, stir-fried (1 cup/124g) 62 cals	0	11
Beet greens: boiled (1 cup/144g) 39 cals	0	12
Beetroot: boiled (2 beets/100g) 44 cals	0	6
Beetroot: fresh (1 beet/81g) 35 cals	0	6
Beetroot: pickled (¼ cup slices/57g) 37 cals	0	1
Beets: Harvard, in butter, sugar and vinegar sauce (½ cup slices/122g) 85 cals	9	5
Borage: fresh (½ cup/44g) 9 cals	0	3
Broad beans: boiled (½ cup/100g) 56 cals (*see also* Legumes & Beans in the Legumes, Nuts and Seeds group)	1	7
Broccoli: boiled (1 cup chopped/156g) 44 cals	1	12
Broccoli: boiled (1 spear/150g) 42 cals	1	11
Broccoli: fresh (1 spear/151g) 42 cals	1	14
Brussels sprouts: boiled (½ cup/78g) 30 cals	0	6

	RISKPOINTS ✗	LIFEPOINTS ✔
Cabbage: Chinese (pak-choi) boiled (1 cup shredded/170g) 20 cals	0	11
Cabbage: Chinese (pak-choi) fresh (1 cup shredded/70g) 9 cals	0	5
Cabbage: red, boiled (1 cup shredded/150g) 32 cals	0	5
Cabbage: red, fresh (1 cup shredded/70g) 19 cals	0	3
Cabbage: savoy, boiled (1 cup shredded/145g) 35 cals	0	7
Cabbage: savoy, fresh (1 cup shredded/70g) 19 cals	0	5
Cabbage: white, boiled (1 cup shredded/150g) 33 cals	1	5
Cabbage: white, fresh (1 cup shredded/70g) 18 cals	0	3
Carrot juice: canned (6 fl oz/184g) 74 cals	0	13
Carrots: baby, fresh (10 medium/100g) 38 cals	1	4
Carrots: boiled (½ cup slices/78g) 35 cals	0	7
Carrots: canned, drained solids (½ can/142g) 33 cals	0	8
Carrots: fresh (1 carrot/72g) 31 cals	0	7
Cauliflower: baked with cheese (1 serving/200g) 226 cals	63	14

	RISKPOINTS ✗	LIFEPOINTS ✓
Cauliflower: boiled (1 cup 1 in pieces/124g) 29 cals	1	7
Cauliflower: fresh (1 cup 1 in pieces/100g) 25 cals	0	6
Celeriac: boiled (1 cup diced/ 150g) 38 cals	0	3
Celeriac: fresh (1 cup/156g) 61 cals	1	6
Celery: boiled (1 cup diced/ 150g) 27 cals	0	5
Celery: fresh (2 stalks/80g) 13 cals	0	3
Celery: soup, cream of (1 cup/8 fl oz/244g) 90 cals	13	3
Chard: Swiss, boiled (1 cup chopped/175g) 35 cals	0	9
Chard: Swiss, fresh (2 leaves/ 96g) 18 cals	0	5
Chicory greens: (escarole or batavia) fresh (1 cup chopped/180g) 41 cals	1	17
Chicory roots: fresh (½ cup 1 in pieces/45g) 33 cals	0	1
Chicory: witloof (most commonly available type; firm, elongated heart), fresh (½ cup/45g) 8 cals	0	1
Chips: *see* Potato chips		
Chives: freeze-dried (¼ cup/ 1g) 2 cals	0	0
Chives: fresh (1 tbsp chopped/3g) 1 cal	0	0

	RISKPOINTS ✗	LIFEPOINTS ✔
Coleslaw (½ cup/60g) 41 cals	3	2
Collards: boiled (1 cup chopped/128g) 35 cals	0	3
Collards: fresh (1 cup chopped/36g) 11 cals	0	1
Corn oil: see Margarines, Oils & Spreads in the Drinks, Desserts, Snacks and Sauces group		
Corn: sweet, canned, creamed (½ cup/128g) 92 cals	1	6
Corn: sweet, boiled (½ cup kernels/82g) 89 cals	2	5
Corn: sweet, canned in brine, drained solids (½ cup/82g) 66 cals	2	4
Corn: sweet, canned with red and green peppers (½ cup/114g) 86 cals	1	5
Corn: sweet, fresh (½ cup cut from cob/77g) 66 cals	2	5
Corn: sweet, on the cob with butter (1 ear/146g) 155 cals	16	9
Cornsalad: see Lamb's lettuce		
Courgettes: boiled (½ cup slices/90g) 14 cals	0	2
Courgettes: fresh (½ cup slices/65g) 9 cals	0	2
Cress: fresh (½ cup/25g) 8 cals	0	3
Cucumber: fresh (½ cup slices/52g) 7 cals	0	1

	RISKPOINTS ✗	LIFEPOINTS ✔
Cucumber, pickled: *see* Dill pickle		
Dandelion greens: fresh (½ cup chopped/28g) 13 cals	0	3
Dill pickle (1 medium/65g) 12 cals	0	0
Dill pickle: sweet (1 medium/ 35g) 41 cals	0	0
Endive: fresh (½ cup chopped/25g) 4 cals	0	2
Escarole: *see* Chicory greens		
Fennel: fresh (1 cup sliced/ 87g) 27 cals	0	3
French beans: *see* Green beans		
French fries: *see* Potato chips		
Garlic: fresh (3 cloves/9g) 13 cals	0	1
Gazpacho soup: canned (1 cup/8 fl oz/244g) 56 cals	5	5
Gherkins: *see* Dill pickle		
Ginger root: fresh (5 slices 1 in diam./11g) 8 cals	0	0
Good King Henry: *see* Lambsquarters		
Green beans: boiled (1 cup/ 125g) 44 cals	0	7
Green beans: canned drained solids (1 can/262g) 52 cals	0	10
Guacamole: *see* Avocado dip		

	RISKPOINTS ✗	LIFEPOINTS ✔
Jerusalem artichokes (½ cup slices/75g) 57 cals	0	4
Jew's ear (pepeao or black mushroom): fresh (½ cup slices/50g) 13 cals	0	2
Kale: boiled (1 cup chopped/ 130g) 42 cals	1	8
Kale: fresh (1 cup chopped/ 67g) 34 cals	1	7
Kohlrabi: boiled (½ cup slices/82g) 24 cals	0	3
Kohlrabi: fresh (½ cup slices/ 70g) 19 cals	0	3
Lamb's lettuce: fresh (1 cup/ 56g) 12 cals	0	4
Lambsquarters (goosefoot): boiled (½ cup chopped/90g) 29 cals	1	9
Lambsquarters: fresh (½ cup/ 50g) 22 cals	1	8
Leek: boiled (1 leek/124g) 38 cals	0	4
Leek: fresh (½ cup chopped/ 52g) 32 cals	0	3
Leek and potato soup: see Vichyssoise		
Lettuce: cos or romaine (4 inner leaves/40g) 6 cals	0	4
Lettuce: butterhead, including round types (4 leaves/30g) 4 cals	0	1

	RISKPOINTS ✗	LIFEPOINTS ✓
Lettuce: iceberg (4 leaves/ 80g) 10 cals	0	3
Lotus root: boiled (5 slices/ 45g) 30 cals	0	2
Mangetout: boiled (½ cup/ 80g) 34 cals	0	5
Mangetout: fresh (½ cup/72g) 30 cals	0	5
Marrow: *see* Squash		
Minestrone soup: canned condensed (½ cup/4 fl oz/ 123g) 84 cals	6	5
Mixed vegetables: *see* Vegetables, mixed		
Mushroom: soup, cream of (1 cup/8 fl oz/248g) 203 cals	59	8
Mushrooms: boiled (½ cup pieces/78g) 21 cals	0	6
Mushrooms: canned, drained solids (½ cup pieces/78g) 19 cals	0	3
Mushrooms: fresh (½ cup pieces/35g) 9 cals	0	3
Mushrooms: shiitake, cooked (4 mushrooms/72g) 40 cals	0	4
Mushrooms: shiitake, dried (4 mushrooms/15g) 44 cals	0	5
Mustard greens: boiled (½ cup chopped/70g) 11 cals	0	5
Mustard greens: fresh (½ cup chopped/28g) 7 cals	0	4

	RISKPOINTS ✗	LIFEPOINTS ✔
Okra: boiled (8 pods/80g) 26 cals	0	5
Olive oil: *see* Margarines, Oils & Spreads in the Drinks, Desserts, Snacks and Sauces group		
Olives: ripe, canned (5 small/16g) 18 cals	4	0
Onion rings: breaded, frozen and reheated (2 rings/20g) 81 cals	13	1
Onions: boiled (½ cup chopped/105g) 46 cals	0	3
Onions: dehydrated flakes (1 tbsp/5g) 16 cals	0	1
Onions: fresh (½ cup chopped/80g) 30 cals	0	2
Onions: sautéed in olive oil (½ cup/115g) 135 cals	25	3
Onion: soup, clear (1 cup/8 fl oz/241g) 58 cals	4	3
Onion: soup, cream of (1 cup/8 fl oz/244g) 107 cals	13	2
Onions: spring, fresh (½ cup chopped/50g) 16 cals	0	3
Pak-choi: *see* Cabbage, Chinese		
Parsley: fresh (½ cup chopped/30g) 11 cals	0	5
Parsnips: boiled (½ cup slices/78g) 63 cals	0	5

	RISKPOINTS ✗	LIFEPOINTS ✔
Parsnips: fresh (½ cup slices/ 67g) 50 cals	0	4
Pea soup: condensed, made up with water (1 cup/8 fl oz/ 250g) 165 cals	14	6
Peas and carrots: frozen, boiled (½ cup/80g) 38 cals	0	6
Peas: canned (½ cup/85g) 59 cals	0	6
Peas: fresh (½ cup/72g) 58 cals	0	8
Peas: fresh, boiled (½ cup/ 80g) 67 cals	0	9
Peas: frozen, boiled (½ cup/ 80g) 67 cals	0	8
Peppers: hot chilli, green, fresh (1 pepper/45g) 18 cals	0	4
Peppers: hot chilli, red, fresh (1 pepper/45g) 18 cals	0	5
Peppers: with rice and lamb filling plus tomato sauce (1 pepper/330g) 289 cals	32	21
Peppers: with vegetable filling and tomato sauce (1 pepper/ 354g) 218 cals	35	19
Peppers: sweet green, boiled (1 pepper/73g) 20 cals	0	3
Peppers: sweet green, fresh (1 pepper/74g) 20 cals	0	3
Peppers: sweet red, fresh (1 pepper/74g) 20 cals	0	5

	RISKPOINTS ✗	LIFEPOINTS ✔
Potato chips: fast food type, fried in beef tallow (1 regular serving/76g) 237 cals	58	5
Potato chips: fast food type, fried in vegetable oil (1 regular serving/76g) 235 cals	30	5
Potato chips: frozen, oven-ready (10 chips/50g) 111 cals	21	3
Potato chips: restaurant type (par-fried then frozen & finished in vegetable oil) (10 chips/50g) 158 cals	20	3
Potato crisps: see Crisps in the Snacks & Sweets section of the Drinks, Desserts, Snacks and Sauces group		

Potato dishes

	RISKPOINTS	LIFEPOINTS
Potato: au gratin, made with butter (1 cup/245g) 323 cals	104	14
Potato: baked, flesh and skin (1 medium potato/202g) 220 cals	0	12
Potato: baked, flesh only (from 1 medium potato/156g) 145 cals	0	7
Potato: baked, skin only (from 1 medium potato/58g) 115 cals	0	7

	RISKPOINTS ✗	LIFEPOINTS ✓
Potato: baked, with baked beans (1 potato/310g) 338 cals	1	20
Potato: baked, with baked beans and margarine (1 potato/315g) 372 cals	11	20
Potato: baked, with butter (1 potato/290g) 256 cals	19	12
Potato: baked, with cheddar cheese and butter (1 potato/330g) 370 cals	61	19
Potato: baked, with cheese sauce (1 potato/296g) 474 cals	124	18
Potato: baked, with cheese sauce and bacon (1 potato/299g) 451 cals	115	21
Potato: baked, with cheese sauce and broccoli (1 potato/339g) 403 cals	96	23
Potato: baked, with cheese sauce and chilli (1 potato/395g) 482 cals	119	28
Potato: baked, with coleslaw (1 potato/290g) 262 cals	4	14
Potato: baked, with cottage cheese (1 potato/310g) 322 cals	10	21
Potato: baked, with margarine (1 potato/290g) 254 cals	9	12

	RISKPOINTS ✗	LIFEPOINTS ✔
Potato: baked, with sour cream and chives (1 potato/302g) 393 cals	56	16
Potato: boiled, flesh only (from 1 medium potato/136g) 118 cals	0	6
Potato: boiled, skin only (from 1 medium potato/34g) 27 cals	0	2
Potato: canned (1 small potato/35g) 21 cals	0	1
Potato: hash browns (½ cup/72g) 151 cals	32	3
Potato: mashed, made from instant granules with milk, water & margarine (1 cup/210g) 166 cals	11	7
Potato: mashed, made with whole milk and margarine (1 cup/210g) 223 cals	22	8
Potato: mashed, made with whole milk, no margarine (1 cup/210g) 162 cals	6	9
Potato: microwaved, flesh and skin (1 medium potato/202g) 212 cals	0	11
Potato: O'Brien, made with milk, onion, breadcrumbs and butter (1 cup/194g) 157 cals	13	8
Potato: scalloped, made with butter (1 cup/245g) 211 cals	50	12

	RISKPOINTS ✗	LIFEPOINTS ✔
Potato flour (1 cup/179g) 628 cals	3	29
Potato pancakes (1 pancake/76g) 207 cals	28	7
Potato salad (½ cup/125g) 179 cals	25	4
Pumpkin: boiled (½ cup mashed/122g) 24 cals	0	3
Pumpkin: canned (½ cup/122g) 41 cals	1	10
Radicchio: fresh (1 cup shredded/40g) 9 cals	0	1
Radishes: fresh (½ cup slices/58g) 10 cals	0	1
Radishes: oriental, fresh (½ cup slices/44g) 8 cals	0	1
Ratatouille: home-made (½ cup/107g) 133 cals	30	3
Runner beans: see Green beans		
Salad: mixed vegetable without dressing, with cheese and egg (1½ cups/217g) 102 cals	22	11
Salad: mixed vegetable without dressing, with prawns (1½ cups/236g) 106 cals	6	19
Salad: mixed vegetable, without dressing (1½ cups/207g) 33 cals	0	9

	RISKPOINTS ✗	LIFEPOINTS ✔
Salsify: boiled (½ cup slices/ 68g) 46 cals	0	3
Sandwich spread: with chopped pickle (1 tbsp/15g) 60 cals	13	0
Sauerkraut: canned, solids & liquid (1 cup/236g) 45 cals	0	9
Shallots: fresh (1 tbsp chopped/10g) 7 cals	0	0
Spinach: boiled (1 cup/180g) 41 cals	1	25
Spinach: canned drained solids (1 cup/214g) 49 cals	2	22
Spinach: fresh (1 cup chopped/56g) 12 cals	0	10
Spinach: frozen, chopped or leaf, boiled (1 cup/190g) 53 cals	0	22
Spinach: soufflé (1 cup/136g) 219 cals	53	18
Spirulina: dried (1 tsp/5g) 15 cals	1	3
Spring greens: see Collards		
Squash: summer varieties (i.e. Chayote, Crookneck), boiled (1 cup slices/180g) 36 cals	1	6
Squash: winter varieties (i.e. Butternut, Acorn), baked (1 cup cubes/205g) 80 cals	3	10
String beans: see Green beans		

	RISKPOINTS ✗	LIFEPOINTS ✔
Swede: boiled (½ cup cubes/ 85g) 33 cals	0	3
Swede: fresh (½ cup cubes/ 70g) 25 cals	0	3
Sweetcorn: see Corn, sweet		
Sweet potato: baked in skin (½ potato/57g) 59 cals	0	6
Sweet potato: boiled without skin (¼ cup mashed/82g) 86 cals	0	7
Tomato juice (6 fl oz/182g) 31 cals	0	6
Tomato ketchup: see Dressings & Sauces in the Drinks, Desserts, Snacks and Sauces group		
Tomato paste: canned (½ cup/131g) 110 cals	2	15
Tomato pureé: canned (½ cup/125g) 51 cals	0	6
Tomato sauce: canned (½ cup/122g) 37 cals	0	5
Tomato soup: condensed, made up with milk (1 cup/8 fl oz/248g) 161 cals	29	11
Tomato soup: condensed, made up with water (1 cup/8 fl oz/244g) 85 cals	4	5
Tomato soup: dehydrated, made up with water (1 pkt/6 fl oz/199g) 78 cals	8	2

	RISKPOINTS ✗	LIFEPOINTS ✔
Tomatoes: green, fresh (1 tomato/123g) 30 cals	0	3
Tomatoes: red, boiled (1 cup/240g) 65 cals	2	8
Tomatoes: red, canned (1 cup/240g) 48 cals	1	7
Tomatoes: red, fresh (1 cup chopped/180g) 38 cals	1	5
Tomatoes: red, fresh (1 tomato/123g) 26 cals	1	3
Tomatoes: sun-dried (8 pieces/16g) 41 cals	1	4
Tomatoes: sun-dried, packed in oil, drained (7 pieces/21g) 45 cals	7	2
Turnip greens: boiled (1 cup chopped/144g) 29 cals	0	16
Turnip greens: fresh (1 cup chopped/55g) 15cals	0	10
Turnips: boiled (½ cup mashed/115g) 21 cals	0	2
Turnips: fresh (½ cup cubes/65g) 18 cals	0	2
Vegetable juice cocktail: canned (6 fl oz/182g) 35 cals	0	7
Vegetable soup: canned, chunky (1 cup/8 fl oz/240g) 122 cals	9	8
Vegetables: mixed, canned, drained solids (1 cup/163g) 77 cals	1	10

	RISKPOINTS ✗	LIFEPOINTS ✔
Vegetables: mixed, frozen, boiled (1 cup/182g) 107 cals	0	11
Vichyssoise (leek and potato soup): (1 cup/8 fl oz/250g) 154 cals	20	7
Water chestnuts: Chinese, canned, solids & liquid (½ cup slices/70g) 35 cals	0	1
Watercress: fresh (½ cup chopped/17g) 2 cals	0	1
Yams: boiled or baked (½ cup cubes/68g) 79 cals	0	3
Yeast extract: fortified with vitamin B12 (1 tsp/5g) 9 cals	0	11
Yellow beans: boiled (1 cup/ 125g) 44 cals	0	6

GROUP 4 – LEGUMES, NUTS AND SEEDS

	RISKPOINTS ✗	LIFEPOINTS ✔
Legumes & Beans		
Adzuki beans: boiled (½ cup/ 115g) 147 cals	0	13
Baked beans: normal (i.e. vegetarian) (½ cup/127g) 118 cals	1	8
Baked beans: on toast (½ can beans and 1 slice toast with butter/238g) 298 cals	22	47
Baked beans: on toast (½ can beans and 1 slice toast, no butter/233g) 263 cals	4	17
Baked beans: with sausages (½ cup/128g) 182 cals	22	9
Black or turtle bean soup (½ cup/4 fl oz/20g) 109 cals	0	9
Black or turtle beans: boiled (½ cup/86g) 114 cals	1	11
Black-eyed beans: boiled (½ cup/86g) 100 cals	1	13
Black-eyed beans: canned (½ cup/120g) 92 cals	1	7
Broad beans: boiled (½ cup/ 85g) 94 cals	0	9
Broad beans: canned (½ cup/ 128g) 91 cals	0	6

	RISKPOINTS ✗	LIFEPOINTS ✔
Broad beans: raw (½ cup/ 75g) 256 cals	2	25
Cannellini beans: boiled (½ cup/90g) 128 cals	1	12
Cannellini beans: canned (½ cup/131g) 153 cals	0	12
Chick peas: boiled (½ cup/ 82g) 134 cals	5	12
Chick peas: brown, boiled (½ cup/77g) 85 cals	2	9
Chick peas: canned (½ cup/ 120g) 143 cals	3	11
Green beans: see Vegetables and Vegetable Products group		
Haricot beans: boiled (½ cup/ 91g) 129 cals	1	12
Haricot beans: canned (½ cup/131g) 148 cals	1	12
Haricot beans: sprouted, boiled (½ cup/85g) 66 cals	1	12
Kidney beans: boiled (½ cup/ 88g) 112 cals	1	12
Kidney beans: canned (½ cup/128g) 104 cals	0	8
Lentils: boiled (½ cup/99g) 115 cals	0	16
Lentils: sprouted, raw (½ cup/ 38g) 40 cals	0	5
Lentils: sprouted, stir-fried (½ cup/38g) 38 cals	0	4

	RISKPOINTS ✗	LIFEPOINTS ✔
Lima beans: boiled (½ cup/ 85g) 105 cals	0	6
Mung beans: boiled (½ cup/ 101g) 106 cals	0	13
Mung beans: sprouted, boiled (1 cup/124g) 26 cals	0	5
Mung beans: sprouted, boiled (½ cup/62g) 13 cals	0	2
Mung beans: sprouted, canned, drained solids (½ cup/62g) 7 cals	0	1
Peanuts: see Nuts & Nut Products		
Peas: split, boiled (½ cup/ 98g) 116 cals	0	9
Pinto beans: boiled (½ cup/ 85g) 116 cals	1	14
Pinto beans: canned (½ cup/ 120g) 94 cals	0	9
Refried beans: canned (½ cup/126g) 135 cals	3	12
Soya beans: boiled (½ cup/ 86g) 149 cals	19	12
Soya beans: sprouted, raw (½ cup/35g) 43 cals	5	6
Soya beans: sprouted, steamed (½ cup/47g) 38 cals	5	4
Soya beans: sprouted, stir-fried (½ cup/47g) 59 cals	8	7

	RISKPOINTS ✗	LIFEPOINTS ✔

Legume & Bean Products

Bacon: meatless (1 rasher/8g) 25 cals	5	3
Bean burger: see Vegetable burger		
Burrito: with beans (2 burritos/217g) 447 cals	51	28
Bean pâté: made with lentils (1 serving/75g) 79 cals	0	11
Carob bar (1 bar/87g) 464 cals	71	17
Carob flavour beverage powder (3 tsp/12g) 45 cals	0	0
Carob flavour beverage powder: made up with milk (1 cup milk + 3 tsp powder/ 256g) 195 cals	38	12
Carob flour (1 tbsp/8g) 31 cals	0	1
Chilli with beans: canned (½ cup/128g) 143 cals	22	10
Dhal: made with mung beans (1 serving/235g) 130 cals	23	13
Falafel (1 patty/17g) 57 cals	7	2
Hummus (½ cup/123g) 210 cals	25	12
Meat substitute: textured vegetable protein (TVP) (1 oz/ 28g) 88 cals	2	21
Miso (1 tbsp/17g) 35 cals	2	2

	RISKPOINTS ✗	LIFEPOINTS ✔
Natto (fermented soybeans) (½ cup/88g) 187 cals	24	13
Sausage: meatless (1 link/ 25g) 64 cals	11	9
Soya bean oil: *see* Margarines, Oils & Spreads in the Drinks, Desserts, Snacks and Sauces group		
Soya milk: (1 cup/240g) 79 cals	11	7
Soya sauce: made from hydrolysed vegetable protein (1 tbsp/18g) 7 cals	0	0
Soya sauce (shoyu): made from soya and wheat (1 tbsp/ 18g) 10 cals	0	1
Soya sauce (tamari): made from soy (1 tbsp/18g) 11 cals	0	1
Tempeh (½ cup/83g) 165 cals	15	14
Tofu: fried (1 piece/13g) 35 cals	6	1
Tofu: fried, made with calcium sulphate (1 piece/13g) 35 cals	6	2
Tofu: fuyu, salted and fermented (1 block/11g) 13 cals	2	0
Tofu: okara (½ cup/61g) 47 cals	2	2
Tofu: raw, firm (¼ block/81g) 117 cals	17	12

	RISKPOINTS ✗	LIFEPOINTS ✔
Tofu: raw, firm, made with calcium sulphate (¼ block/ 81g) 117 cals	17	15
Tofu: raw, regular (¼ block/ 116g) 88 cals	13	8
Tofu: raw, regular, made with calcium sulphate (¼ block/ 116g) 88 cals	13	11
TVP: *see* Meat substitute		
Vegetable burger (1 patty/ 92g) 108 cals	11	9
Vegetable burger in bun, with lettuce, tomato & ketchup (1 burger/176g) 243 cals	17	17

Nuts & Nut Products

	RISKPOINTS ✗	LIFEPOINTS ✔
Almond: butter (1 tbsp/16g) 101 cals	23	3
Almond oil: *see* Margarines, Oils & Spreads in the Drinks, Desserts, Snacks and Sauces group		
Almonds: dried, blanched (24 kernels/28g) 166 cals	37	5
Almonds: dried, unblanched (24 kernels/28g) 167 cals	37	6
Almonds: dry-roasted, unblanched (24 kernels/28g) 167 cals	36	6
Almonds: ground (1 oz/28g) 168 cals	36	5

	RISKPOINTS ✗	LIFEPOINTS ✓
Almonds: honey-roasted, unblanched (24 kernels/28g) 168 cals	35	5
Almonds: oil-roasted, blanched (24 kernels/28g) 174 cals	40	5
Almonds: oil-roasted, unblanched (22 kernels/28g) 176 cals	40	7
Almonds: toasted, unblanched (24 kernels/28g) 167 cals	36	6
Brazil nuts: dried (6–8 kernels/28g) 186 cals	47	5
Cashew: nut butter, plain (1 tbsp/16g) 94 cals	19	2
Cashews: dry-roasted (1 oz/ 28g) 163 cals	32	5
Cashews: oil-roasted (1 oz/ 28g) 164 cals	34	5
Chestnuts: Chinese, boiled and steamed (1 oz/28g) 43 cals	0	2
Chestnuts: Chinese, dried (1 oz/28g) 103 cals	1	4
Chestnuts: Chinese, roasted (1 oz/28g) 68 cals	0	3
Chestnuts: sweet, boiled and steamed (1 oz/28g) 37 cals	0	2
Chestnuts: sweet, roasted (1 oz/28g) 70 cals	1	3

	RISKPOINTS ✗	LIFEPOINTS ✔
Coconut: cream, canned (liquid expressed from grated meat) (1 tbsp/19g) 36 cals	22	0
Coconut: cream, fresh (liquid expressed from grated meat (1 tbsp/15g) 50 cals	34	0
Coconut: creamed (1 oz/28g) 194 cals	130	2
Coconut: desiccated, unsweetened (1 oz/28g) 187 cals	121	2
Coconut: meat, raw (1 cup shredded or grated/80g) 283 cals	178	5
Coconut: meat, raw (1 piece/45g) 159 cals	100	2
Coconut: milk (1 tbsp/15g) 3 cals	0	0
Filberts: see Hazelnuts		
Ginkgo nuts: dried (1 oz/28g) 99 cals	1	6
Ginkgo nuts: raw (1 oz/28g) 52 cals	1	3
Hazelnut oil: see Margarines, Oils & Spreads in the Drinks, Desserts, Snacks and Sauces group		
Hazelnuts: dried, blanched (1 oz/28g) 191 cals	47	5
Hazelnuts: dried, unblanched (1 oz/28g) 179 cals	44	5

	RISKPOINTS ✗	LIFEPOINTS ✔
Hazelnuts: dry-roasted, unblanched (1 oz/28g) 188 cals	47	5
Hazelnuts: oil-roasted, unblanched (1 oz/28g) 187 cals	45	5
Hickory nuts: dried (1 oz/28g) 187 cals	45	5
Macadamia nuts: dried (1 oz/28g) 199 cals	52	3
Macadamia nuts: oil-roasted (10–12 kernels/28g) 204 cals	54	2
Mixed nuts with peanuts: dry-roasted (10–12 kernels/28g) 169 cals	36	5
Mixed nuts with peanuts: oil-roasted (1 oz/28g) 175 cals	39	6
Mixed nuts without peanuts: oil-roasted (1 oz/28g) 175 cals	39	5
Peanut butter: chunky (2 tbsp/32g) 188 cals	39	7
Peanut butter: smooth (2 tbsp/32g) 188 cals	39	6
Peanut butter: sandwich with banana (1 sandwich/201g) 433 cals	51	21
Peanut butter: sandwich with jam (1 sandwich/127g) 425 cals	50	15

	RISKPOINTS ✗	LIFEPOINTS ✔
Peanuts: boiled (½ cup/32g) 102 cals	17	4
Peanuts: dry-roasted (1 oz/ 28g) 164 cals	34	7
Peanuts: oil-roasted (1 oz/ 28g) 163 cals	34	8
Peanuts: raw (1 oz/28g) 159 cals	34	10
Pecans: dried (1 oz/28g) 189 cals	48	4
Pecans: dry-roasted (20 halves/28g) 187 cals	45	3
Pecans: oil-roasted (20 halves/28g) 195 cals/	50	3
Pine nuts: dried (15 kernels/ 28g) 146 cals	35	6
Pistachios: dried (47 kernels/ 28g) 164 cals	34	6
Pistachios: dry-roasted (47 kernels/28g) 172 cals	37	4
Pumpkin & squash seeds: dried (142 kernels/28g) 154 cals	32	7
Pumpkin & squash seeds: roasted (142 kernels/28g) 148 cals	29	7
Sesame oil: see Margarines, Oils & Spreads in the Drinks, Desserts, Snacks and Sauces group		

	RISKPOINTS ✗	LIFEPOINTS ✔
Sesame seed paste (1 tbsp/16g) 95 cals	20	6
Sesame seeds: whole, dried (1 tbsp/9g) 52 cals	11	4
Sesame seeds: whole, roasted or toasted (1 tbsp/9g) 51 cals	10	4
Sunflower oil: see Margarines, Oils & Spreads in the Drinks, Desserts, Snacks and Sauces group		
Sunflower seed butter (1 tbsp/16g) 93 cals	19	5
Sunflower seeds: dried (1 oz/28g) 162 cals	35	13
Sunflower seeds: dry-roasted (1 oz/28g) 165 cals	35	9
Sunflower seeds: oil-roasted (1 oz/28g) 175 cals	40	9
Sunflower seeds: toasted (1 oz/28g) 176 cals	40	9
Tahini: made from raw & stone-ground sesame kernels (1 tbsp/15g) 86 cals	18	5
Tahini: made from roasted or toasted sesame kernels, the most common type (1 tbsp/15g) 89 cals	20	5
Tahini: made from unroasted sesame kernels, with non-chemical removal of seed coat (1 tbsp/14g) 85 cals	19	5

	RISKPOINTS ✗	LIFEPOINTS ✓
Walnut oil: *see* Margarines, Oils & Spreads in the Drinks, Desserts, Snacks and Sauces group		
Walnuts: dried (1 oz/28g) 182 cals	43	4

GROUP 5 – MEAT, FISH AND DAIRY PRODUCTS

	RISKPOINTS ✗	LIFEPOINTS ✓

MEAT – Beef

	RISKPOINTS ✗	LIFEPOINTS ✓
All cuts: trimmed, lean & fat, cooked without additional fat (3 oz/85g) 259 cals	54	20
All cuts: trimmed, lean, cooked without additional fat (3 oz/85g) 184 cals	24	22
Beef-cured pastrami (2 slices/ 56g) 198 cals	44	10
Beef dripping (1 tbsp/13g) 115 cals	47	0
Beef jerky: chopped and pressed (1 oz/28g) 96 cals	12	12
Beef stick: *see* Meat-based snack sticks		
Beerwurst (beer salami): *see* Sausages & Luncheon Meats		
Bologna: *see* Sausages & Luncheon Meats		
Brisket: lean and fat, braised (3 oz/85g) 327 cals	78	18
Brisket: lean only, braised (3 oz/85g) 206 cals	29	21
Burgers: cheeseburger (1 large double patty with condiments & vegetables/258g) 704 cals	132	36

	RISKPOINTS ✗	LIFEPOINTS ✔
Burgers: cheeseburger (1 large single patty with bacon & condiments/195g) 608 cals	121	32
Burgers: cheeseburger (1 large single patty with condiments & vegetables/219g) 563 cals	112	31
Burgers: cheeseburger (1 large single patty with ham, condiments & vegetables/254g) 744 cals	158	39
Burgers: cheeseburger (1 large single patty, plain/185g) 609 cals	111	35
Burgers: hamburger (1 large double patty with condiments & vegetables/226g) 540 cals	78	33
Burgers: hamburger (1 large single patty, plain/137g) 426 cals	62	26
Burgers: hamburger (1 large single patty, with condiments & vegetables/218g) 512 cals	78	30
Burgers: vegetable burger: see Legume & Bean Products in the Legumes, Nuts and Seeds group		
Chilli con carne (1 cup/253g) 256 cals	25	25
Corned beef: canned (1 slice/21g) 53 cals	9	3
Corned beef: jellied loaf (2 slices/56g) 87 cals	11	8

	RISKPOINTS ✗	LIFEPOINTS ✓
Cured dried beef (1 oz/28g) 47 cals	3	7
Cured thin-sliced beef (1 oz/28 g) 50 cals	3	7
Frankfurter: beef (1 frankfurter/57g) 180 cals	51	7
Hotdog: in roll (141g) 365 cals	42	18
Hotdog: without roll (98g) 242 cals	38	13
Meat-based snack sticks (salami-style): smoked (1 stick/20g) 109 cals	30	3
Mince: extra lean, baked, medium rare (3 oz/85g) 213 cals	40	17
Mince: extra lean, grilled, medium rare (3 oz/85g) 218 cals	40	19
Mince: extra lean, pan-fried, medium rare (3 oz/85g) 217 cals	41	19
Mince: lean, baked, medium rare (3 oz/85g) 228 cals	45	17
Mince: lean, grilled, medium rare (3 oz/85g) 231 cals	46	19
Mince: lean, pan-fried, medium rare (3 oz/85g) 234 cals	47	19
Mince: regular, baked, medium rare (3 oz/85g) 244 cals	52	18

	RISKPOINTS ✗	LIFEPOINTS ✔
Mince: regular, grilled, medium rare (3 oz/85g) 246 cals	51	19
Mince: regular, pan-fried, medium rare (3 oz/85g) 260 cals	56	19
Porterhouse steak: lean & fat, grilled (3 oz/85g) 259 cals	56	19
Porterhouse steak: lean, grilled (3 oz/85g) 185 cals	27	21
Rib steak: lean & fat, grilled (3 oz/85g) 275	65	18
Roast beef: sandwich, plain (139g) 346 cals	34	23
Roast beef: sandwich, with cheese (176g) 473 cals	67	32
Roast beef: sandwich, on French bread (216g) 410 cals	53	28
Rump steak: lean & fat, grilled (3 oz/85g) 190 cals	26	20
Rump steak: lean, grilled (3 oz/85g) 162 cals	16	20
Sirloin steak: lean & fat, grilled (3 oz/85g) 208 cals	35	21
Sirloin steak: lean, grilled (3 oz/85g) 166 cals	17	23
Soup, beef & noodles (1 cup/ 8 fl oz/244g) 83 cals	17	5
Soup: beef & tomato with noodles (1 cup/8 fl oz/244g) 139 cals	23	5

	RISKPOINTS ✗	LIFEPOINTS ✔
Soup: beef & vegetable (1 cup/8 fl oz/244g) 78 cals	6	5
Soup: beef broth, bouillon & consommé (1 cup/8 fl oz/ 241g) 29 cals	0	2
Soup: oxtail (1 cup/8 fl oz/ 253g) 71 cals	9	2
Steak & kidney pie (1 serving/ 250g) 808 cals	166	25
Steak: sandwich (204g) 459 cals	35	32
Stew: home-made (1 cup/ 252g) 222 cals	13	22
Stroganoff (1 serving/349g) 603 cals	150	35
T-bone steak: lean & fat, grilled (3 oz/85g) 253 cals	54	19
T-bone steak: lean, grilled (3 oz/85g) 182 cals	26	21
Topside: lean & fat, grilled (3 oz/85g) 247 cals	50	20
Topside: lean & fat, roasted (3 oz/85g) 282 cals	64	18
Topside: lean, grilled (3 oz/ 85g) 179 cals	23	22
Topside: lean, roasted (3 oz/ 85g) 189 cals	27	20

Chicken

Breast meat and skin: fried in batter (3 oz/85g) 221 cals	28	13

	RISKPOINTS ✗	LIFEPOINTS ✔
Breast meat and skin: roasted (3 oz/85g) 167 cals	16	15
Breast meat and skin: stewed (3 oz/85g) 156 cals	15	10
Breast meat only: fried (3 oz/85g) 159 cals	10	17
Breast meat only: roasted (3 oz/85g) 140 cals	7	15
Breast meat only: stewed (3 oz/85g) 128 cals	6	11
Chicken fat (1 tbsp/12g) 115 cals	31	0
Chicken meat: canned, boned with stock (½ can/71g) 117 cals	14	8
Chicken roll: light meat (1 slice/1 oz/28g) 45 cals	5	2
Chicken salad spread (1 tbsp/13g) 26 cals	4	0
Chicken paste: canned (1 tbsp/13g) 25 cals	3	1
Chicken stock cubes: dry (1 cube/5g) 10 cals	0	0
Drumstick meat and skin: fried in batter (1 drumstick/72g) 193 cals	28	9
Drumstick meat and skin: roasted (1 drumstick/52g) 112 cals	14	7

	RISKPOINTS ✗	LIFEPOINTS ✔
Drumstick meat and skin: stewed (1 drumstick/57g) 116 cals	15	6
Drumstick meat only: fried (1 drumstick/42g) 82 cals	8	6
Drumstick meat only: roasted (1 drumstick/44g) 76 cals	6	6
Drumstick meat only: stewed (1 drumstick/46g) 78 cals	6	6
Fast food: boneless pieces, breaded and fried, plain (6 pieces/102g) 290 cals	44	12
Fast food: boneless pieces, breaded and fried, with barbecue sauce (6 pieces/130g) 330 cals	44	13
Fast food: boneless pieces, breaded and fried, with honey (6 pieces/115g) 329 cals	43	12
Fast food: boneless pieces, breaded and fried, with mustard sauce (6 pieces/130g) 322 cals	47	13
Fast food: boneless pieces, breaded and fried, with sweet and sour sauce (6 pieces/130g) 346 cals	44	13
Fast food: breast or wing, light meat, breaded and fried (2 pieces/163g) 494 cals	73	22

	RISKPOINTS ✗	LIFEPOINTS ✔
Fast food: drumstick or thigh, dark meat, breaded and fried (2 pieces/148g) 431 cals	66	20
Frankfurter: chicken (1 frankfurter/45g) 116 cals	21	4
Giblets: fried (3 oz/85g) 235 cals	28	43
Giblets: simmered (3oz/85g) 133 cals	10	32
Gizzard: simmered (½ cup/70g) 107 cals	6	16
Heart: simmered (½ cup/70g) 130 cals	13	25
Liver: simmered (½ cup/70g) 110 cals	9	34
Meat and skin: fried in batter (3 oz/85g) 246 cals	36	11
Meat and skin: roasted (3 oz/85g) 203 cals	28	13
Meat and skin: stewed (3 oz/85g) 186 cals	26	10
Meat only: fried (3 oz/85g) 186 cals	19	15
Meat only: roasted (3 oz/85g) 162 cals	15	14
Meat only: stewed (3 oz/85g) 150 cals	14	11
Salad: chicken and vegetable, with dressing (1½ cups/263g) 280 cals	43	16

	RISKPOINTS ✗	LIFEPOINTS ✔
Salad: chicken and vegetable, without dressing (1½ cups/218g) 105 cals	5	15
Sandwiches: chicken fillet, plain (1 sandwich/182g) 515 cals	73	19
Sandwiches: chicken fillet, with cheese (1 sandwich/228g) 632 cals	96	27
Soup: chicken and mushroom (1 cup/8 fl oz/244g) 132 cals	22	4
Soup: chicken and vegetables (1 cup/8 fl oz/240g) 166 cals	12	9
Soup: chicken noodle, canned chunky, ready-to-serve (1 cup/8 fl oz/240g) 175 cals	15	9
Soup: cream of chicken (1 cup/8 fl oz/248g) 191 cals	34	9
Sweet and sour chicken (1 serving/453g) 626 cals	41	25
Wing meat and skin: fried in batter (1 wing/49g) 159 cals	26	5
Wing meat and skin: roasted (1 wing/34g) 99 cals	16	4
Wing meat and skin: stewed (1 wing/40g) 100 cals	16	4
Wing meat only: fried (1 wing/20g) 42 cals	4	3

	RISKPOINTS ✗	LIFEPOINTS ✔
Wing meat only: roasted (1 wing/21g) 43 cals	4	3
Wing meat only: stewed (1 wing/24g) 43 cals	4	2

Duck

Meat and skin: roasted (3 oz/85g) 286 cals	61	11
Meat only: roasted (3 oz/85g) 171 cals	26	14

Game

Grouse: roasted meat only (3 oz/85g) 147 cals	11	16
Hare: stewed, meat only (3 oz/85g) 163 cals	20	8
Partridge: roasted meat only (3 oz/85g) 180 cals	15	8
Pheasant: roasted meat only (3 oz/85g) 181 cals	19	11
Wild boar: roasted (3 oz/85g) 136 cals	9	8
Wild rabbit: stewed (3 oz/85g) 147 cals	7	9

Goose

Meat & skin: roasted (3 oz/85g) 259 cals	46	12
Meat only: roasted (3 oz/85g) 202 cals	29	15

	RISKPOINTS ✗	LIFEPOINTS ✔
Pâté de foie gras (goose liver pâté): smoked (1 oz/28g) 131 cals	31	11

Gravy

	RISKPOINTS ✗	LIFEPOINTS ✔
Au jus (made with meat juices) (½ cup/119g) 19 cals	0	3
Beef (½ cup/116g) 61 cals	10	3
Chicken (½ cup/119g) 94 cals	16	2
Granules: dehydrated then prepared with water (½ cup/129g) 37 cals	3	1
Turkey (½ cup/118g) 60 cals	6	3

Lamb

British	RISKPOINTS ✗	LIFEPOINTS ✔
All cuts: lean & fat, cooked (3 oz/85g) 250 cals	56	20
All cuts: lean only, cooked (3 oz/85g) 175 cals	21	21
Chop: lean & fat, grilled (3 oz/85g) 307 cals	80	19
Chop: lean & fat, roasted (3 oz/85g) 305 cals	81	18
Chop: lean only, grilled (3 oz/85g) 200 cals	29	21
Chop: lean only, roasted (3 oz/85g) 197 cals	30	19

	RISKPOINTS ✗	LIFEPOINTS ✔
Leg: lean & fat, roasted (3 oz/ 85g) 219 cals	43	20
Leg: lean only, roasted (3 oz/ 85g) 162 cals	17	21
Moussaka (1 serving/225g) 439 cals	79	24
Scotch broth (1 cup/8 fl oz/ 241g) 80 cals	16	5
Shepherd's pie (1 serving/ 225g) 268 cals	42	21
New Zealand		
All cuts: lean & fat, cooked (3 oz/85g) 259 cals	70	20
All cuts: lean only, cooked (3 oz/85g) 175 cals	24	22

Pork

	RISKPOINTS ✗	LIFEPOINTS ✔
Bacon: back, grilled (3 oz/ 85g) 157 cals	18	18
Bacon: gammon, grilled, pan-fried or roasted (3 oz/85g) 490 cals	111	22
Bacon: meatless (i.e. vegetarian): *see* Legume & Bean Products in the Legumes, Nuts and Seeds group		
Bacon: streaky, grilled, pan-fried or roasted (3 oz/85g) 390 cals	81	24

	RISKPOINTS ✗	LIFEPOINTS ✔
Bacon sandwich: (1 sandwich with 2 slices bacon/101g) 225 cals	19	17
Banger: *see* Sausage		
Blade: lean & fat, braised (3 oz/85g) 271 cals	50	19
Blade: lean & fat, grilled (3 oz/85g) 220 cals	37	19
Blade, lean & fat, roasted (3 oz/85g) 229 cals	44	17
Blade: lean only, braised (3 oz/85g) 232 cals	35	20
Blade: lean only, grilled (3 oz/85g) 193 cals	28	20
Blade: lean only, roasted (3 oz/85g) 197 cals	33	23
BLT sandwich (bacon, lettuce and tomato): (1 sandwich/ 151g) 265 cals	34	15
Brains: braised (3 oz/85g) 117 cals	20	11
Brawn: pork (1 slice/1 oz/ 28g) 60 cals	11	3
Chops: lean & fat, braised (3 oz/85g) 213 cals	37	15
Chops: lean & fat, grilled (3 oz/85g) 224 cals	36	20
Chops: lean & fat, pan-fried (3 oz/85g) 225 cals	40	17
Chops, lean & fat, roasted (3 oz/85g) 217 cals	37	17

	RISKPOINTS ✗	LIFEPOINTS ✔
Chops: lean only, braised (3 oz/85g) 175 cals	23	15
Chops: lean only, grilled (3 oz/85g) 186 cals	22	21
Chops: lean only, pan-fried (3 oz/85g) 185 cals	25	18
Chops: lean only, roasted (3 oz/85g) 190 cals	27	18
Ears: simmered (1 ear/111g) 184 cals	32	5
Ham, cured: chopped, canned (1 slice/21g) 50 cals	9	3
Ham, cured: croquettes, grilled (1 croquette/59g) 203 cals	49	7
Ham, cured: lean & fat, roasted (3 oz/85g) 207 cals	38	14
Ham, cured: lean only, roasted (3 oz/85g) 133 cals	11	17
Ham & cheese sandwich: (1 sandwich/146g) 352 cals	48	20
Ham, egg & cheese sandwich: (1 sandwich/143g) 347 cals	55	24
Ham patties: grilled (1 patty/59g) 203 vals	49	7
Heart: braised (1 heart/129g) 191 cals	16	38
Kidneys: braised (3 oz/85g) 128 cals	9	32
Lard (1 tbsp/12g) 115 cals	37	0

	RISKPOINTS ✗	LIFEPOINTS ✓
Leg: lean & fat, roasted (3 oz/ 85g) 232 cals	41	17
Leg: lean only, roasted (3 oz/ 85g) 179 cals	21	18
Liver: braised (3 oz/85g) 140 cals	9	45
Liver sausage: see Sausages & Luncheon Meats		
Liverwurst: see Sausages & Luncheon Meats		
Loin: lean & fat, braised (3 oz/85g) 203 cals	32	15
Loin: lean & fat, grilled (3 oz/ 85g) 206 cals	33	18
Loin: lean & fat, roasted (3 oz/85g) 211 cals	34	19
Loin: lean only, braised (3 oz/ 85g) 173 cals	21	16
Loin: lean only, grilled (3 oz/ 85g) 179 cals	23	19
Loin: lean only, roasted (3 oz/ 85g) 178 cals	22	20
Lungs: braised (3 oz/85g) 84 cals	6	20
Mince: cooked without additional fat (3 oz/85g) 252 cals	49	16
Pork pie (1 individual pie/ 210g) 730 cals	121	34
Pork scratchings (1 oz/28g) 155 cals	24	4

	RISKPOINTS ✗	LIFEPOINTS ✔
Sausage: fresh, cooked without additional fat (1 sausage/27g) 100 cals	21	6
Sausage meat: cooked (1 oz/ 28g) 103 cals	22	6
Sausage roll (1 roll/55g) 263 cals	58	2
Shoulder: lean & fat, roasted (3 oz/85g) 248 cals	50	16
Shoulder: lean only, roasted (3 oz/85g) 196 cals	30	18
Soup: ham & split pea, canned, chunky (1 cup/8 fl oz/240g) 185 cals	11	10
Spareribs: lean & fat, braised (3 oz/85g) 337 cals	70	19
Tongue: braised (3 oz/85g) 230 cals	41	23
Trotters: pickled (1 oz/28g) 58 cals	11	2

Rabbit

All cuts: roasted (3 oz/85g) 167 cals	17	21
All cuts: stewed (3 oz/85g) 175 cals	17	20
Wild: see Game		

Sausages & Luncheon Meats

Beef luncheon meat: loaf (1 slice/28g) 87 cals	23	7

	RISKPOINTS ✗	LIFEPOINTS ✔
Beef luncheon meat: thin-sliced (1 slice/4g) 7 cals	0	1
Beerwurst (beer salami): pork (1 slice/6g) 14 cals	2	0
Beerwurst (beer salami): pork (1 slice/23g) 76 cals	22	3
Berliner (1 slice/23g) 53 cals	10	4
Black pudding: *see* Blood sausage		
Blood sausage or blood pudding (1 slice/25g) 95 cals	25	3
Bockwurst (1 sausage/65g) 200 cals	49	9
Bologna: beef (1 slice/1 oz/ 28g) 88 cals	25	3
Bologna: beef & pork (1 slice/ 23g) 73 cals	18	3
Bologna: pork (1 slice/23g) 57 cals	11	3
Bratwurst (1 sausage/85g) 256 cals	59	13
Braunschweiger (liver sausage): smoked (1 slice/ 18g) 65 cals	14	12
Braunschweiger: cured pork (1 slice/18g) 65 cals	14	12
Brawn: *see* Pork		
Brotwurst (1 sausage/70g) 226 cals	52	12

	RISKPOINTS ✗	LIFEPOINTS ✔
Chicken liver pâté: canned (1 tbsp/13g) 26 cals	4	9
Chorizo (1 sausage/60g) 273 cals	64	15
Cured beef luncheon meat: jellied (1 slice/28g) 31 cals	2	9
Cured ham: chopped, canned (1 slice/21g) 50 cals	9	3
Cured ham: minced & pressed (1 slice/21g) 55 cals	11	3
Goose liver pâté: *see* Pâté de foie gras		
Ham & cheese spread (1 tbsp/15g) 37 cals	9	2
Ham luncheon meat: sliced (1 slice/28g) 52 cals	7	5
Ham salad spread (1 tbsp/15g) 32 cals	5	1
Ham: chopped, not canned (1 slice/21g) 48 cals	9	3
Ham: chopped, spiced, canned (1 slice/21g) 50 cals	9	3
Italian sausage: cooked (1 sausage/67g) 216 cals	45	13
Liver cheese: cured pressed pork (1 slice/38g) 116 cals	25	22
Liver sausage (liverwurst): pork (1 slice/18g) 59 cals	14	11
Luncheon meat sandwiches: with French bread (1 sandwich/228g) 456 cals	51	30

	RISKPOINTS ✗	LIFEPOINTS ✔
Mixed pork & beef sausage: cooked (1 sausage/13g) 51 cals	12	1
Mortadella (1 slice/15g) 47 cals	10	2
Pâté de foie gras: canned, smoked (1 tbsp/13g) 60 cals	14	6
Pâté: mixed meat or unspecified meat (1 tbsp/13g) 41 cals	9	3
Peppered luncheon meat (1 slice/28g) 42 cals	4	5
Pepperoni (1 slice/5g) 27 cals	6	1
Pickle & pimento luncheon meat: made with pork (1 slice/28g) 74 cals	16	4
Picnic luncheon meat (1 slice/28g) 66 cals	12	4
Polish-style sausage (1 sausage/227g) 740 cals	175	33
Pork & beef luncheon meat (1 slice/28g) 100 cals	24	4
Pork & beef sandwich spread: (1 tbsp/15g) 35 cals	6	1
Pork & olive luncheon meat (1 slice/28g) 67 cals	12	4
Pork chipolatas: cooked (1 sausage/13g) 48 cals	10	2
Pork luncheon meat: canned (1 slice/21g) 70 cals	16	2

	RISKPOINTS ✗	LIFEPOINTS ✔
Smoked pork sausage (1 sausage/68g) 265 cals	57	15
Thuringer (1 slice/23g) 77 cals	20	7
Turkey & ham luncheon meat (1 slice/28g) 36 cals	3	3
Vienna sausage: canned (1 sausage/16g) 45 cals	11	1

Turkey

Boneless turkey meat: roasted (3 oz/85g) 132 cals	12	15
Breast: meat & skin, prebasted & roasted (3 oz/85g) 107 cals	7	11
Breast: meat & skin, roasted (3 oz/85g) 161 cals	15	12
Dark meat: roasted (3 oz/85g) 159 cals	25	13
Giblets: simmered with some giblet fat (3 oz/85g) 142 cals	10	32
Leg: meat & skin, roasted (3 oz/85g) 177 cals	20	13
Liver: simmered (3 oz/85g) 144 cals	12	35
Meat: canned with stock (3 oz/85g) 139 cals	14	11
Meat & skin: roasted (3 oz/85g) 177 cals	20	12
Meat only: roasted (3 oz/85g) 145 cals	10	13

	RISKPOINTS ✗	LIFEPOINTS ✔
Mince: cooked, no additional fat (1 patty/82g) 193 cals	26	11
Patties: breaded, battered & fried (1 patty/3 oz/85g) 266 cals	42	9
Soup: canned, chunky (1 cup/ 8 fl oz/236g) 135 cals	11	16
Thigh: meat & skin, prebasted & roasted (3 oz/85g) 133 cals	18	10
Turkey roll: made from white & dark meat (3 oz/85g) 127 cals	14	10
Turkey sticks: breaded, battered & fried (1 stick/2¼ oz/64g) 179 cals	27	6
White meat: roasted (3 oz/ 85g) 133 cals	6	13
Wing: meat & skin, roasted (1 wing/186g) 426 cals	57	26

Veal

	RISKPOINTS ✗	LIFEPOINTS ✔
Lean & fat meat: braised (3 oz/85g) 179 cals	24	20
Lean & fat meat: breaded & pan-fried (3 oz/85g) 194 cals	19	19
Lean & fat meat: pan-fried, not breaded (3 oz/85g) 179 cals	31	21
Lean & fat meat: roasted (3 oz/85g) 136 cals	17	17

	RISKPOINTS ✗	LIFEPOINTS ✔
Lean only: braised (3 oz/85g) 173 cals	18	20
Lean only: breaded & pan-fried (3 oz/85g) 175 cals	13	20
Lean only: pan-fried, not breaded (3 oz/85g) 156 cals	9	22
Lean only: roasted (3 oz/85g) 128 cals	12	18
Mince: grilled (3 oz/85g) 146 cals	19	17

Venison

Roasted (3 oz/85g) 134 cals	7	14

FISH & SEAFOOD

Note: Throughout this section, 'moist heat' includes cooking methods such as steaming, stewing and inclusion in soups and sauces. 'Dry heat' includes methods such as grilling and baking.

Abalone: fried (3 oz/85g) 161 cals	14	10
Anchovy: canned in oil, drained solids (5 anchovies/ 20g) 42 cals	4	5
Bass: freshwater, cooked dry heat (1 fillet/62g) 91 cals	7	11

	RISKPOINTS ✗	LIFEPOINTS ✔
Bass, sea: cooked dry heat (1 fillet/101g) 125 cals	6	10
Bass: striped, cooked dry heat (1 fillet/124g) 154 cals	9	18
Bream: see Carp		
Burbot: cooked dry heat (1 fillet/90g) 104 cals	2	14
Carp: cooked dry heat (1 fillet/170g) 275 cals	30	25
Catfish: breaded & fried (1 fillet/87g) 199 cals	28	13
Caviar: black & red granular (1 tbsp/16g) 40 cals	7	11
Clam: breaded & fried (10 small clams/94g) 190 cals	26	22
Clam: canned, drained solids (3 oz/85g) 126 cals	4	27
Clam: canned, with liquid (3 oz/85g) 2 cals	0	8
Clam: cooked moist heat (10 small clams/94g) 139 cals	4	28
Cod liver oil (1 tbsp/13g) 123 cals	34	0
Cod: canned, solids & liquid (1 can/312g) 328 cals	6	30
Cod: cooked dry heat (1 fillet/180g) 189 cals	3	22
Cod: dried & salted (3 oz/85g) 247 cals	5	29

	RISKPOINTS ✗	LIFEPOINTS ✔
Crab cakes: (1 cake/60g) 93 cals	11	15
Crab: canned (3 oz/85g) 84 cals	2	11
Crab: cooked moist heat (3 oz/85g) 87 cals	3	19
Crayfish: wild, cooked moist heat (3 oz/85g) 75 calls	2	14
Cuttlefish: cooked moist heat (3 oz/85g) 134 cals	2	31
Eel: cooked dry heat (1 fillet/159g) 375 cals	59	24
Fish & chips: 1 fillet plaice fried in batter & 1 standard portion chips fried in vegetable oil (256g) 737 cals	111	19
Fish fillet: battered, or breaded & fried (1 fillet/91g) 211 cals	27	12
Fish fingers (1 finger/28g) 76 cals	8	4
Fish pie (1 serving/200g) 256 cals	36	17
Flatfish (flounder & sole species): cooked dry heat (1 fillet/127g) 149 cals	4	18
Flounder: see Flatfish		
Gefilte fish: sweet recipe (1 piece/42g) 35 cals	1	3
Grouper: cooked dry heat (1 fillet/202g) 238 cals	6	21

	RISKPOINTS ✗	LIFEPOINTS ✔
Haddock: cooked dry heat (1 fillet/150g) 168 cals	3	23
Haddock: smoked (3 oz/85g) 99 cals	2	14
Halibut: Atlantic, cooked dry heat (½ fillet/159g) 223 cals	11	28
Halibut: Greenland, cooked dry heat (½ fillet/159g) 380 cals	70	18
Herring: cooked dry heat (1 fillet/143g) 290 cals	41	25
Herring: kippered (1 fillet/40g) 87 cals	12	13
Herring: pickled (1 piece/15g) 39 cals	6	3
Kedgeree (1 serving/115g) 174 cals	20	14
Kipper: see Herring		
Ling: cooked dry heat (1 fillet/151g) 168 cals	3	20
Lobster: cooked moist heat (3 oz/85g) 83 cals	1	14
Lox: see Salmon, smoked		
Mackerel: Atlantic, cooked dry heat (1 fillet/88g) 231 cals	39	20
Mackerel: canned, drained solids (1 can/190g) 296 cals	29	33
Mackerel: king, cooked dry heat (1 fillet/308g) 413 cals	19	48

	RISKPOINTS ✗	LIFEPOINTS ✔
Monkfish: cooked dry heat (3 oz/85g) 82 cals	4	9
Mullet: cooked dry heat (1 fillet/93g) 140 cals	11	12
Mussel: cooked moist heat (3 oz/85g) 146 cals	9	24
Oyster: breaded & fried (6 medium oysters/88g) 173 cals	27	23
Oyster: canned (3 oz/85g) 59 cals	5	22
Oyster: stew, canned, condensed (1 cup/8 fl oz/ 246g) 118 cals	37	18
Oyster: wild, cooked moist heat (6 medium oysters/42g) 58 cals	5	21
Perch: cooked dry heat (1 fillet/46g) 54 cals	1	8
Perch, ocean: cooked dry heat (1 fillet/50g) 61 cals	2	7
Pike: cooked dry heat (1 fillet/ 124g) 148 cals	4	23
Pike: northern, cooked dry heat (½ fillet/155g) 175 cals	3	22
Pollack: cooked dry heat (½ fillet/151g) 178 cals	4	23
Prawns: breaded & fried (4 large prawns/30g) 73 cals	9	5
Prawns: canned (3 oz/85g) 102 cals	4	11

	RISKPOINTS ✗	LIFEPOINTS ✔
Prawns: cooked moist heat (4 large prawns/22g) 22 cals	0	3
Prawn salad sandwich with mayonnaise (1 sandwich/148g) 263 cals	29	16
Rainbow trout: see Trout		
Roe: cooked dry heat (3 oz/85g) 173 cals	17	25
Salmon: Atlantic, wild, cooked dry heat (½ fillet/154g) 280 cals	31	39
Salmon: canned, drained solids with bone (3 oz/85g) 130 cals	15	11
Salmon: cooked dry heat (½ fillet/155g) 335 cals	42	26
Salmon: pink, canned solids with bone & liquid (3 oz/85g) 118 cals	12	18
Salmon: pink, cooked dry heat (½ fillet/124g) 185 cals	13	23
Salmon: smoked (3 oz/85g) 99 cals	9	14
Salmon: smoked (lox) (3 oz/85g) 99 cals	9	14
Sardine: Atlantic, canned in oil, drained solids with bone (2 sardines/24g) 50 cals	6	11
Sardine: Atlantic, canned in oil, drained solids with bone (1 can/92g) 191 cals	26	22

	RISKPOINTS ✗	LIFEPOINTS ✔
Sardine: Pacific, canned in tomato sauce, drained solids with bone (2 sardines/76g) 135 cals	22	17
Sardine: Pacific, canned in tomato sauce, drained solids with bone (1 can/370g) 659 cals	110	51
Scallop: breaded & fried (2 large scallops/31g) 67 cals	8	3
Scampi: breaded & fried (6 pieces/164g) 454 cals	62	16
Seafood salad: vegetable and pasta, without dressing (1½ cups/417g) 379 cals	52	24
Shad: cooked dry heat (1 fillet/144g) 363 cals	63	24
Shark: batter-dipped & fried (3 oz/85g) 194 cals	29	11
Smelt: cooked dry heat (3 oz/85g) 105 cals	6	15
Snapper: cooked dry heat (1 fillet/170g) 218 cals	7	21
Sole: *see* Flatfish		
Spiny lobster: cooked moist heat (1 lobster/163g) 233 cals	7	30
Squid: fried (3 oz/85g) 149 cals	15	12
Sturgeon: cooked dry heat (3 oz/85g) 115 cals	11	18

	RISKPOINTS ✗	LIFEPOINTS ✔
Sturgeon: smoked (3 oz/85g) 147 cals	9	20
Swordfish: cooked dry heat (3 oz/85g) 132 cals	10	18
Tomato bisque: canned, condensed (1 cup/8 fl oz/ 257g) 247 cals	12	8
Trout: cooked dry heat (1 fillet/62g) 118 cals	13	17
Trout: rainbow, cooked dry heat (1 fillet/71g) 120 cals	12	17
Trout, sea: cooked dry heat (1 fillet/186g) 247 cals	21	25
Tuna: canned in oil, drained solids (1 can/171g) 339 cals	35	28
Tuna: canned in oil, drained solids (3 oz/85g) 168 cals	17	19
Tuna: canned in water, drained solids (1 can/165g) 191 cals	3	28
Tuna: canned in water, drained solids (3 oz/85g) 99 cals	1	20
Tuna salad (3 oz/85g) 159 cals	19	11
Tuna: salad sandwich on French bread (256g) 584 cals	69	29
Turbot: cooked dry heat (½ fillet/159g) 194 cals	15	20
Turbot, sea: see Ling		

	RISKPOINTS ✗	LIFEPOINTS ✔
Whelk: cooked moist heat (3 oz/85g) 234 cals	1	26
Whitefish: cooked dry heat (1 fillet/154g) 265 cals	28	23
Whitefish: smoked (3 oz/85g) 92 cals	1	15
Whiting: cooked dry heat (1 fillet/72g) 83 cals	3	13

DAIRY
Butter

	RISKPOINTS ✗	LIFEPOINTS ✔
Butter (1 pat/5g) 36 cals	18	0
Butter blends: *see* Margarine, Oils & Spreads		
Ghee: clarified butter (1 tbsp/ 13g) 112 cals	46	0

Cheese

	RISKPOINTS ✗	LIFEPOINTS ✔
Brie (1 oz/28g) 93 cals	36	5
Camembert (1 oz/28g) 84 cals	32	5
Cheddar (1 oz/28g) 114 cals	42	5
Cheddar & pickle sandwich (105g) 293 cals	53	15
Cheddar & tomato sandwich (150g) 292 cals	53	17
Cheese & ham spread: *see* Sausages & Luncheon Meats		
Cheese fondue (1 serving/ 80g) 229 cals	77	12

	RISKPOINTS ✗	LIFEPOINTS ✔
Cheese soufflé (1 cup/136g) 343 cals	86	16
Cheshire (1 oz/28g) 108 cals	40	5
Cottage: creamed, large or small curd (1 oz/28g) 29 cals	5	2
Cottage: creamed, large or small curd (4 oz/113g) 117 cals	24	8
Cottage: 2% fat (1 oz/28g) 25 cals	2	2
Cottage: 2% fat (4 oz/113g) 101 cals	10	9
Cream cheese (1 oz/28g) 98 cals	46	1
Edam (1 oz/28g) 100 cals	36	6
Feta (1 oz/28g) 74 cals	31	7
Fontina (1 oz/28g) 109 cals	40	7
Gjetost (1 oz/28g) 130 cals	40	7
Goat: hard (1 oz/28g) 128 cals	52	7
Goat: semi-soft (1 oz/28g) 103 cals	43	3
Goat: soft (1 oz/28g) 76 cals	30	3
Gouda (1 oz/28g) 100 cals	36	6
Gruyère (1 oz/28g) 116 cals	39	7
Mozzarella: part skimmed milk (1 oz/28g) 71 cals	21	4
Mozzarella: whole milk (1 oz/28g) 79 cals	27	3

	RISKPOINTS ✗	LIFEPOINTS ✔
Neufchatel (1 oz/28g) 73 cals	31	1
Parmesan: grated (1 oz/28g) 128 cals	40	8
Parmesan: grated (1 tbsp/5g)	7	1
Parmesan (1 oz/28g) 110 cals	34	7
Port Salut (1 oz/28g) 98 cals	35	5
Processed (1 oz/28g) 93 cals	32	5
Provolone (1 oz/28g) 98 cals	35	6
Ricotta: part skimmed milk (¼ cup/62g) 86 cals	22	5
Ricotta: whole milk (¼ cup/62g) 108 cals	38	5
Romano (1 oz/28g) 108 cals	35	6
Roquefort (1 oz/28g) 103 cals	40	5
Swiss (1 oz/28g) 105 cals	37	7
Swiss: pasteurised, processed (1 oz/28g) 90 cals	32	6
Tilsit: whole milk (1 oz/28g) 95 cals	35	6
Welsh rarebit (1 serving/60g) 219 cals	62	8

Cream

Cream: double (1 tbsp/15g) 37 cals	17	0
Cream: single (1 tbsp/15g) 29 cals	13	0

	RISKPOINTS ✗	LIFEPOINTS ✓
Cream: sour (1 tbsp/12g) 26 cals	11	0
Cream: substitute, non-dairy powder (1 tsp/2g) 11 cals	4	0
Cream: whipped, topping, pressurised (1 tbsp/3g) 8 cals	3	0
Cream: whipping, heavy (1 tbsp/15g) 52 cals	25	0
Cream: whipping, light (1 tbsp/15g) 44 cals	21	0
Dessert topping: non-dairy, powdered (1 tbsp/1g) 8 cals	3	0
Dessert topping: non-dairy, pressurised (1 tbsp/4g) 11 cals	5	0

Eggs (chicken's unless otherwise stated)

	RISKPOINTS ✗	LIFEPOINTS ✓
Dried (1 tbsp/5g) 30 cals	5	3
Dried: powder (¼ cup sifted/ 27g) 102 cals	0	9
Dried: yolk only (1 tbsp/4g) 27 cals	6	2
Duck egg: raw (1 egg/70g) 130 cals	24	17
Egg & cheese sandwich (146g) 340 cals	49	20
Egg, cress & mayonnaise sandwich (145g) 284 cals	36	17
Egg custard: baked (½ cup/ 141g) 148 cals	24	8

	RISKPOINTS ✗	LIFEPOINTS ✔
Egg mayonnaise sandwich (135g) 335 cals	48	15
Egg substitute: powder (0.35 oz/9g) 44 cals	3	4
Fried (1 large egg/46g) 92 cals	17	6
Goose egg: raw (1 egg/144g) 267 cals	47	27
Hard-boiled (1 large egg/50g) 78 cals	13	7
Omelette (1 large egg/59g) 90 cals	16	6
Omelette (2 eggs/120g) 182 cals	34	12
Poached (1 large egg/50g) 75 cals	12	6
Quail egg: raw (1 egg/9g) 14 cals	2	1
Quiche Lorraine (1 serving/115g) 450 cals	107	15
Raw: white only (1 large egg/33g) 17 cals	0	1
Raw: yolk & white (1 large egg/50g) 75 cals	12	7
Raw: yolk only (1 large egg/16g) 59 cals	12	5
Scotch egg (1 egg/115g) 321 cals	67	13
Scrambled (1 egg/60g) 100 cals	18	7

	RISKPOINTS ✗	LIFEPOINTS ✓

Milk (cow's unless otherwise stated)

	RISKPOINTS ✗	LIFEPOINTS ✓
Buttermilk: cultured from skimmed milk (1 cup/245g) 99 cals	10	10
Buttermilk: dried (1 tbsp/6g) 25 cals	1	3
Condensed milk: canned, sweetened (1 fl oz/38g) 123 cals	15	3
Dried: skimmed milk, non-fat solids (¼ cup/30g) 109 cals	1	15
Dried: whole milk (¼ cup/32g) 159 cals	40	12
Evaporated: canned, unsweetened (1 fl oz/31g) 42 cals	10	2
Ewe's milk (1 cup/245g) 264 cals	84	22
Goat's milk (1 cup/244g) 168 cals	48	9
Malted milk beverage (1 cup milk + ¾ oz powder/265g) 236 cals	44	17
Malted milk: dry powder (¾ oz/2–3 tsp/21g) 87 cals	6	5
Malted milk: dry powder, chocolate (¾ oz/2–3 tsp/21g) 79 cals	3	2
Milkshake: thick chocolate (300g) 356 cals	37	16

	RISKPOINTS ✗	LIFEPOINTS ✓
Milkshake: thick vanilla (313g) 350 cals	44	19
Semi-skimmed milk (1 cup/ 244g) 136 cals	22	14
Skimmed milk (1 cup/244g) 86 cals	2	12
Whole milk (1 cup/244g) 157 cals	41	12

Yogurt

Low-fat (½ carton/113g) 72 cals	8	8
Low-fat: with fruit (½ carton/ 113g) 115 cals	5	7
Skimmed milk (½ carton/ 113g) 63 cals	0	9
Whole milk (½ carton/113g) 69 cals	17	5

GROUP 6 – DRINKS, DESSERTS, SNACKS AND SAUCES

	RISKPOINTS ✗	LIFEPOINTS ✔

Drinks

	RISKPOINTS	LIFEPOINTS
Apple juice: *see* Fruit and Fruit Juices group		
Apricot nectar: *see* Fruit and Fruit Juices group		
Cappucino (1 cup/212g) 86 cals	33	1
Carbonated soft drink: non-cola, e.g. lemonade (12 fl oz can/368g) 147 cals	0	0
Carrot juice: *see* Vegetables and Vegetable Products group		
Cherry juice: *see* Fruit and Fruit Juices group		
Cocoa: home-made from hot milk (1 cup/8 fl oz/250g) 218 cals	42	14
Coffee: ground (6 fl oz/177g) 4 cals	0	0
Coffee: instant (1 rounded tsp/2g) 4 cals	0	0
Coffee: instant decaffeinated (1 rounded tsp/2g) 4 cals	0	0
Coffee substitute: cereal grain beverage powder (1 tsp/2g) 9 cals	0	0

	RISKPOINTS ✗	LIFEPOINTS ✔
Cola (12 fl oz can/370g) 152 cals	0	0
Cola: low-calorie (12 fl oz can/355g) 4 cals	0	0
Cranberry juice: *see* Fruit and Fruit Juices group		
Cranberry juice cocktail: *see* Fruit and Fruit Juices group		
Egg nog (½ cup/4 fl oz/127g) 171 cals	42	7
Ginger ale (12 fl oz can/366g) 124 cals	0	0
Grape juice: *see* Fruit and Fruit Juices group		
Grapefruit juice: *see* Fruit and Fruit Juices group		
Lemon juice: *see* Fruit and Fruit Juices group		
Lemonade: *see* Carbonated soft drink		
Lime Juice: *see* Fruit and Fruit Juices group		
Malted milk: with added nutrients prepared with milk (1 cup/8 fl oz milk plus 3 heaped tsp powder/265g) 231 cals	40	34
Malted milk: with no added nutrients prepared with milk (1 cup/8 fl oz milk plus 3 heaped tsp powder/265g) 236 cals	44	17

	RISKPOINTS ✗	LIFEPOINTS ✓
Milkshake: chocolate (10 fl oz/283g) 359 cals	49	16
Milkshake: vanilla (10 fl oz/283g) 314 cals	39	14
Orange juice: *see* Fruit and Fruit Juices group		
Passion-fruit juice: *see* Fruit and Fruit Juices group		
Peach nectar: *see* Fruit and Fruit Juices group		
Pear nectar: *see* Fruit and Fruit Juices group		
Pineapple juice: *see* Fruit and Fruite Juices group		
Prune juice: *see* Fruit and Fruit Juices group		
Tangerine juice: *see* Fruit and Fruit Juices group		
Tea: herb (6 fl oz/178g) 2 cals	0	0
Tea: no milk or sugar (6 fl oz/178g) 2 cals	0	0
Tea: with milk, no sugar (1 cup/8 fl oz/238g)	12	3
Tea: with milk, one sugar (1 cup/8 fl oz/242g) 56 cals	12	3
Tea: with milk, two sugars (1 cup/8 fl oz/246g) 71 cals	12	3
Tomato juice: *see* Vegetables and Vegetable Products group		

	RISKPOINTS ✗	LIFEPOINTS ✔
Tonic water (12 fl oz can/ 366g) 124 cals	0	0
Vegetable juice cocktail: see Vegetables and Vegetable Products group		
Vinegar: cider (1 tbsp/15g) 2 cals	0	0
Water: mineral, unflavoured (1 cup/8 fl oz/237g)	0	0

Biscuits & Cookies

	RISKPOINTS ✗	LIFEPOINTS ✔
Arrowroot biscuits (1 biscuit/ 2g) 11 cals	0	0
Brownie (large/56g) 227 cals	22	4
Chocolate chip cookie: soft-type (1 biscuit/15g) 69 cals	9	0
Chocolate wafers (1 wafer/ 6g) 26 cals	2	0
Coconut macaroon: home-made (1 macaroon/24g) 97 cals	20	0
Custard cream (1 biscuit/14g) 72 cals	15	0
Digestive: chocolate-coated (large/14g) 68 cals	11	1
Digestive: plain (large/7g) 30 cals	1	0
Fig roll (1 biscuit/16g) 56 cals	2	1
Gingernut (1 biscuit/7g) 29 cals	1	0

	RISKPOINTS ✗	LIFEPOINTS ✓
Peanut butter cookie (1 biscuit/15g) 72 cals	8	1
Shortbread: plain (1 biscuit/8g) 40 cals	4	0

Cakes, Pastries & Puddings

As you will see, none of the following can fairly be described as 'health food'. But if you really want to know the damage, here's the awful truth . . .

Angelfood cake (1 serving/53g) 142 cals	0	2
Apple crumble (1 serving/115g) 239 cals	21	3
Apple pie (1 serving/155g) 411 cals	48	5
Apple strudel (1 serving/71g) 195 cals	19	2
Bread pudding (½ cup/126g) 212 cals	21	7
Bread & butter pudding (1 serving/115g) 183 cals	34	6
Carrot cake: with cream cheese icing (1 serving/111g) 484 cals	73	6
Carrot cake: without icing (1 serving/70g) 239 cals	27	7
Cheesecake (1 serving/80g) 257 cals	69	4

	RISKPOINTS ✗	LIFEPOINTS ✔
Cherry pie (1 serving/125g) 325 cals	34	2
Chocolate cake: with chocolate icing (1 serving/64g) 235 cals	26	3
Chocolate pudding: made with whole milk (½ cup/142g) 158 cals	22	6
Christmas pudding (1 serving/115g) 350 cals	46	6
Coffee cake: buttercream-filled with chocolate icing (1 serving/90g) 298 cals	24	5
Crème caramel: made with whole milk (½ cup/133g) 150 cals	18	5
Cream puff (1 shell/66g) 239 cals	42	6
Danish pastry (65g) 262 cals	36	7
Doughnut: ring, glazed (1 medium/60g) 242 cals	34	6
Doughnut: ring, plain (1 medium/47g) 198 cals	26	3
Doughnut: creme filling (1 doughnut/85g) 307 cals	52	7
Doughnut: jam filling (1 doughnut/85g) 289 cals	39	6
Eclair: custard-filled with chocolate glaze (1 eclair/100g) 262 cals	39	7
Filo pastry (1 sheet/19g) 57 cals	2	2

	RISKPOINTS ✗	LIFEPOINTS ✔
Fruit cake (1 small serving/ 43g) 139 cals	9	1
Fruit jelly (½ cup/106g) 73 cals	0	1
Gingerbread cake (1 serving/ 74g) 263 cals	30	5
Ice cream cones: 'sugar' or wafer-type (1 cone/4g) 17 cals	0	0
Icing: chocolate, made with butter (1 serving/50g) 200 cals	26	0
Icing: chocolate, made with margarine (1 serving/50g) 201 cals	14	0
Icing: glaze (1 serving/27g) 97 cals	5	0
Icing: vanilla, made with butter (1 serving/48g) 165 cals	9	0
Icing: vanilla, made with margarine (1 serving/48g) 194 cals	12	0
Jam tarts (1 tart/40g) 154 cals	17	1
Jelly (1 packet/14g) 38 cals	4	0
Lemon meringue pie (1 serving/113g) 303 cals	24	5
Madeira cake (1 serving/74g) 291 cals	48	2

	RISKPOINTS ✗	LIFEPOINTS ✔
Marble cake: no icing (1 serving/73g) 253 cals	31	3
Mince pies (1 individual pie/ 50g) 218 cals	29	2
Pastry: puff, baked (1 oz/28g) 158 cals	27	2
Pastry: short-crust, baked (1 serving/23g) 121 cals	19	2
Pecan pie (1 serving/122g) 503 cals	67	8
Pineapple upside-down cake (1 serving/115g) 367 cals	34	7
Pound cake: made with butter (1 serving/53g) 229 cals	57	4
Pumpkin pie (1 serving/155g) 316 cals	36	9
Rice pudding: canned (1 can/ 5 oz/142g) 231 cals	26	4
Sponge cake (1 serving/38g) 110 cals	2	3
Suet pudding (1 serving/ 115g) 383 cals	87	5
Tapioca pudding: made with whole milk (½ cup/141g) 161 cals	19	5
Treacle tart (1 serving/115g) 427 cals	47	4
Trifle (1 serving/115g) 184 cals	24	4
Yellow cake: with chocolate icing (1 serving/64g) 243 cals	27	3

	RISKPOINTS ✗	LIFEPOINTS ✔

Dressings & Sauces

	RISKPOINTS ✗	LIFEPOINTS ✔
Barbecue sauce (½ cup/4 fl oz/125g) 94 cals	5	3
Bolognese sauce (¾ cup/6 fl oz/200g) 278 cals	54	21
Cheddar cheese sauce: made with milk (½ cup/4 fl oz/140g) 154 cals	35	9
Hollandaise sauce: made with milk & butter (1 cup/8 fl oz/254g) 703 cals	313	9
Ketchup (1 tbsp/15g) 16 cals	2	0
Mayonnaise: made without dairy products (i.e. vegan) (1 tbsp/14g) 67 cals	16	0
Mayonnaise: made with soya bean oil (1 tbsp/13g) 99 cals	27	0
Mayonnaise: made with soya bean & safflower oil (1 tbsp/13g) 99 cals	27	0
Mornay sauce (½ cup/168g) 242 cals	64	15
Mustard: plain (1 tbsp/17g) 40 cals	6	2
Mustard: prepared with cream (1 tbsp/17g) 28 cals	9	0
Pickle: sweet (1 tbsp/15g) 20 cals	2	0
Salad dressing: blue cheese (1 tbsp/15g) 77 cals	20	0

	RISKPOINTS ✗	LIFEPOINTS ✓
Salad dressing: French, ready made (1 tbsp/14g) 88 cals	24	0
Salad dressing: French, low-fat, ready made (1 tbsp/16g) 22 cals	2	0
Salad dressing: Italian, low-fat (1 tbsp/15g) 16 cals	3	0
Salad dressing: thousand island (1 tbsp/15g) 59 cals	13	0
Salad dressing: thousand island, low-fat (1 tbsp/15g) 24 cals	4	0
Salad dressing: oil & vinegar (1 tbsp/15g) 70 cals	19	0
Sesame seed dressing (1 tbsp/15g) 68 cals	17	0
Sweet & sour sauce (½ cup/4 fl oz/156g) 147 cals	0	2
Tartar sauce (1 tbsp/20g) 61 cals	12	0
Teriyaki sauce (1 tbsp/18g) 15 cals	0	0
White sauce: made with milk (½ cup/4 fl oz/131g) 119 cals	23	7

Snacks & Sweets

Banana chips (1 oz/28g) 147 cals	61	1
Burgers: see Beef in the Meat, Fish and Dairy Products group		

	RISKPOINTS ✗	LIFEPOINTS ✔
Butterscotch topping (2 tbsp/ 41g) 103 cals	0	0
Caramel cookie bar (1 bar/ 57g) 272 cals	33	3
Caramel topping: see Butterscotch topping		
Carob cookie (1 bar/3 oz/ 87g) 464 cals	71	17
Chewing gum (1 stick/3g) 10 cals	0	0
Chips: see Potato chips in the Vegetables and Vegetable Products Group		
Chocolate: after-dinner mints (2 pieces/8g) 29 cals	4	0
Chocolate: baking chocolate, unsweetened (1 square/1 oz/ 28g) 148 cals	69	3
Chocolate: caramels in milk chocolate (1 packet/55g) 261 cals	29	4
Chocolate: fudge (1 piece/ 17g) 65 cals	6	0
Chocolate: milk (1 bar/44g) 226 cals	60	4
Chocolate: milk chocolate-coated peanuts (10 nuts/40g) 208 cals	43	5
Chocolate: milk chocolate-coated raisins (10 raisins/ 10g) 39 cals	6	0

	RISKPOINTS ✗	LIFEPOINTS ✔
Chocolate: plain (1 oz/28g) 143 cals	42	1
Chocolate: plain, bitter, regular (1 oz/28g) 135 cals	37	1
Chocolate: plain, dark, made with butter (1 oz/28g) 135 cals	37	1
Chocolate: snack bar (1 bar/ 2.1 oz/60g) 251 cals	35	4
Chocolate: wafer bar (1 bar/ 1.6oz/4g) 235 cals	57	4
Crisps: barbecue flavoured (1 oz/28g) 139 cals	22	4
Crisps: made from dried potatoes, lower fat (1 oz/28g) 142 cals	18	3
Crisps: made from dried potatoes, plain (1 oz/28g) 158 cals	27	2
Crisps: plain (1 oz/28g) 152 cals	24	3
Crisps: sour cream & onion flavour (1 oz/28g) 151 cals	24	5
Fish & chips: see Fish in the Meat, Fish and Dairy Products group		
Fish fillet: see Fish in the Meat, Fish and Dairy Products group		
Fish fingers: see Fish in the Meat, Fish and Dairy Products group		

	RISKPOINTS ✗	LIFEPOINTS ✔
Fruit leather bar (1 bar/23g) 81 cals	6	0
Honey: strained or extracted (1 tbsp/21g) 64 cals	0	0
Ice cream: chocolate (1 serving/66g) 143 cals	40	4
Ice cream: strawberry (1 serving/66g) 127 cals	13	3
Ice cream: vanilla, rich (1 serving/74g) 178 cals	55	3
Ice cream: vanilla, soft-serve (1 serving/86g) 185 cals	48	5
Ice cream: vanilla, standard (1 serving/66g) 133 cals	40	3
Ice cream: yogurt, soft-serve (1 serving/72g) 114 cals	18	4
Ices: sorbet, made with water & fruit only (1 serving/96g) 75 cals	0	0
Jams & preserves: all varieties (1 tbsp/20g) 48 cals	0	0
Jellybeans (10 small/11g) 40 cals	5	0
Lemon curd (1 tbsp/20g) 58 cals	10	0
Marmalade: orange (1 tbsp/ 20g) 49 cals	5	0
Marshmallows (1 regular/7g) 23 cals	2	0
Molasses: blackstrap (1 tbsp/ 20g) 47 cals	0	5

	RISKPOINTS ✗	LIFEPOINTS ✔
Molasses: light (1 tbsp/20g) 53 cals	2	1
Muesli bar (1 bar/24g) 115 cals	12	2
Nachos: with cheese (6–8 nachos/113g) 346 cals	58	14
Nachos: with cheese, beans, ground beef and peppers (6–8 nachos/255g) 569 cals	93	25
Nuts: see Legumes, Nuts and Seeds group		
Pancakes: see Cooked Breakfast Foods in the Cereals,Grains and Pasta group		
Peanut bar (1 bar/45g) 235 cals	37	6
Peanut brittle (1 oz/28g) 128 cals	13	3
Pizza: see Breads in the Cereals, Grains and Pasta group		
Popcorn: air-popped (1 cup/ 8g) 31 cals	0	1
Popcorn: caramel-coated (1 cup/35g) 152 cals	11	1
Popcorn: cheese-flavour (1 cup/11g) 58 cals	9	1
Popcorn: oil-popped (1 cup/ 11g) 55 cals	7	1

	RISKPOINTS ✗	LIFEPOINTS ✓
Potato sticks (1 oz/28g) 148 cals	24	3
Pretzels: hard, salted (10 twists/60g) 229 cals	5	11
Sesame crunch: e.g. sesame snaps (1 oz/28g) 147 cals	23	7
Sugar: brown types (1 tsp/4g) 15 cals	3	0
Sugar: white, granulated (1 tsp/4g) 15 cals	3	0
Sugar: icing (1 tbsp unsifted/ 8g) 31 cals	6	0
Syrup: chocolate (2 tbsp/1 fl oz/37g) 82 cals	1	0
Syrup: corn, high-fructose (1 tbsp/19g) 53 cals	0	0
Syrup: golden (1 tbsp/20g) 57 cals	4	0
Syrup: malt (1 tbsp/24g) 76 cals	9	2
Syrup: maple (1 tbsp/20g) 52 cals	4	0
Taco salad (1½ cups/198g) 279 cals	51	16
Taco salad with chilli con carne (1½ cups/261g) 290 cals	45	22
Toffee (1 piece/12g) 65 cals	18	0
Tortilla chips: nacho-flavour (1 oz/28g) 141 cals	18	2

	RISKPOINTS ✗	LIFEPOINTS ✔
Tortilla chips: plain (1 oz/ 28g) 142 cals	18	2
Trail mix (1 oz/28g) 131 cals	20	5
Welsh rarebit: *see* Cheese in the Meat, Fish and Dairy Products group		

Margarines, Oils & Spreads

For butter and ghee see Dairy in the Meat, Fish and Dairy Products group.

Almond oil (1 tbsp/13.6g) 120 cals	34	0
Corn oil: salad or cooking (1 tbsp/13.6g) 120 cals	34	0
Grapeseed oil (1 tbsp/13.6g) 120 cals	34	0
Hazelnut oil (1 tbsp/13.6g) 120 cals	34	0
Margarine/butter: 60% corn oil & 40% butter (1 tsp/5g) 36 cals	10	0
Margarine: hard, made with hydrogenated corn oil (1 tsp/ 4g) 34 cals	9	0
Margarine: hard, made with hydrogenated soya bean oil (1 tsp/4g) 34 cals	9	0

	RISKPOINTS ✗	LIFEPOINTS ✔
Margarine: hard, made with hydrogenated sunflower & soya bean oils (1 tsp/4g) 34 cals	9	0
Margarine: low-fat (approx. 40%) made with hydrogenated soya bean oil (1 tsp/4g) 17 cals	4	0
Margarine: soft, made with hydrogenated or non-hydrogenated corn oil (1 tsp/4g) 34 cals	9	0
Margarine: soft, made with hydrogenated or non-hydrogenated soya bean oil (1 tsp/4g) 34 cals	9	0
Margarine: soft, made with hydrogenated or non-hydrogenated sunflower oil (1 tsp/4g) 34 cals	9	0
Margarine: soft, made with unspecified oils (1 tsp/4g) 34 cals	9	0
Olive oil: salad or cooking (1 tbsp/13.5g) 119 cals	33	0
Peanut oil: salad or cooking (1 tbsp/13g) 119 cals	33	0
Sesame oil: salad or cooking (1 tbsp/13.6g) 120 cals	34	0
Soya bean oil: salad or cooking (1 tbsp/13.6g) 120 cals	34	0

	RISKPOINTS ✗	LIFEPOINTS ✔
Sunflower oil: salad or cooking (1 tbsp/13.6g) 120 cals	34	0
Vegetable shortening: made with hydrogenated soya bean & palm oils (1 tbsp/12g) 113 cals	32	0
Walnut oil (1 tbsp/13.6g) 120 cals	34	0
Wheatgerm oil (1 tbsp/13.6g) 120 cals	34	0

Herbs & Spices

Allspice: ground (1 tsp/1g) 5 cals	0	0
Anise seed (1 tsp/2g) 7 cals	0	0
Basil: dried (1 tsp/1g) 4 cals	0	0
Basil: fresh (5 leaves/2g) 1 cal	0	0
Bay leaf: crumbled (1 tsp/1g) 2 cals	0	0
Caraway seed (1 tsp/2g) 7 cals	0	0
Cardamom: ground (1 tsp/2g) 6 cals	0	0
Celery seed (1 tsp/2g) 8 cals	1	0
Chervil: dried (1 tsp/1g) 1 cal	0	0
Chilli powder (1 tsp/2g) 8 cals	1	1
Cinnamon: ground (1 tsp/2g) 6 cals	0	1

	RISKPOINTS ✗	LIFEPOINTS ✔
Cloves: ground (1 tsp/2g) 7 cals	1	0
Coriander: dried (1 tsp/1g) 2 cals	0	0
Coriander: fresh (¼ cup/4g) 1 cal	0	0
Coriander seed (1 tsp/1g) 5 cals	0	0
Cumin seed (1 tsp/2g) 8 cals	1	1
Curry powder (1 tsp/2g) 7 cals	0	0
Dill seed (1 tsp/2g) 6 cals	0	0
Dill weed: dried (1 tsp/1g) 3 cals	0	0
Dill weed: fresh (5 sprigs/1g) 1 cal	0	0
Fennel seed (1 tsp/2g) 7 cals	0	0
Fenugreek seed (1 tsp/3g) 12 cals	0	1
Garlic powder (1 tsp/2g) 9 cals	0	0
Ginger: ground (1 tsp/1g) 6 cals	0	0
Mace: ground (1 tsp/1g) 8 cals	1	0
Marjoram: dried (1 tsp/1g) 2 cals	0	0
Mustard seed: yellow (1 tsp/3g) 15 cals	2	0
Nutmeg: ground (1 tsp/2g) 12 cals	4	0

	RISKPOINTS ✗	LIFEPOINTS ✔
Onion powder (1 tsp/2g) 7 cals	0	0
Oregano: dried (1 tsp/1g) 5 cals	0	0
Paprika (1 tsp/2g) 6 cals	0	1
Parsley: dried (1 tsp/1g) 1 cal	0	0
Parsley: fresh (10 sprigs/10g) 4 cals	0	1
Pepper: black (1 tsp/2g) 5 cals	0	0
Pepper: red or cayenne (1 tsp/1g) 6 cals	0	0
Pepper: white (1 tsp/2g) 7 cals	0	0
Poppy seed (1 tsp/2g) 15 cals	3	1
Rosemary: dried (1 tsp/1g) 4 cals	0	0
Saffron (1 tsp/1g) 2 cals	0	0
Sage: dried (1 tsp/1g) 5 cals	0	0
Tarragon: dried (1 tsp/1g) 5 cals	0	0
Thyme: dried (1 tsp/1g) 4 cals	0	1
Turmeric: ground (1tsp/2g) 8 cals	0	0

INDEX

Index

Index